THROUGH THE

Best Wishes

George W Jones

THROUGH THE TUNNEL

George W Jones

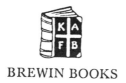

BREWIN BOOKS

First published by
Brewin Books, Studley, Warwickshire, B80 7LG
in 1994

© George W Jones

ISBN 1 85858 037 4

British Library Cataloguing in Publication Data
A Catalogue record for this book is available from the British Library

Typeset in Times by Avon Dataset Ltd, Bidford on Avon, Warks, B50 4JH
Printed in Great Britain by Supaprint, Redditch, Worcs.

Day One

It was a miserable day in early April, cold ,wet and very windy. The wind coming from the south east over an unbroken landscape blew relentlessly without gusting, so there was no momentary respite from the coldness of the drizzle on my unprotected face. I was on my way.

It was a beginning that might never have happened, a beginning with a potentially disastrous preamble that should have left me feeling exhausted and tense, but to my relief I felt fit, fresh and confident. The weather could have been a little more auspicious, but the biting cold only added to my resolve. At last it had begun.

Kreiss, Reiss and on to Wick. The place names repeated themselves in my mind like the refrain of a well loved nursery rhyme. As I fairly bounced along the unfamiliar route, searched my limited horizon for a glimpse of any road signs which bore the well rehearsed names of places I was to pass through. Wick was my destination on this first day, and by the time I reached it, I should have walked seventeen miles and nearly two percent of my total journey in a little over four hours.

This was a beginning. But this beginning was the flowering of an idea that had germinated six months before, and its nurturing and growth had been fraught with such difficulties that I had, at times, wondered how such a simple and single-minded plan could become so complex .

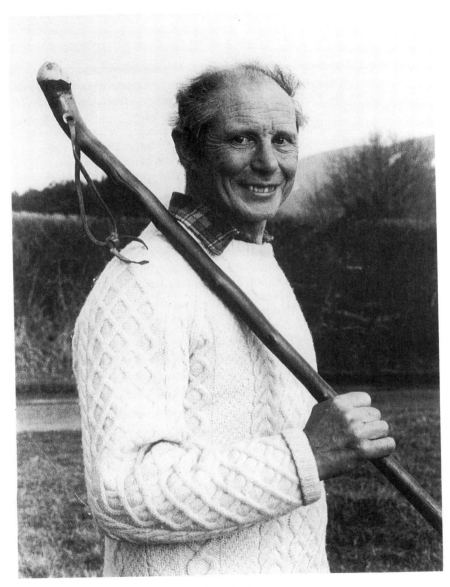

The Author

2

The Birth of an idea

It started in October 1990 when I was told about three children aged between 3 and 6 years who were facing the inevitability of blindness. It was a story that made me feel at once helpless, and deeply sad. I have lived with encroaching blindness for much of my adult life and finally, at the age of 65, I had to accept that I was, then, to all intents and purposes, blind. But to think of the same inexorable disease destroying the sight of small children was something I found difficult; surely something could be done to help them?

The sight-destroying disease which affects me, those children, and many others is that of Retinitis Pigmentosa (R.P.). It is a hereditary disorder, which results in the eventual destruction of the retina of the eye, the part which reflects the image it sees before transferring it to the brain. I have belonged to the Birmingham branch of the Retinitis Pigmentosa society for many years, and have been involved in research programmes and fund-raising, desperately hoping that a cure can be found to prevent others from losing their sight as I have. It was at one of the R.P. society meetings that I heard about these three children; just three more in a long line of tragedies caused by this disease.

On the Monday following this particular meeting, I was doing what I enjoy most, walking on the Long Mynd, near my home in South Shropshire. It occurred to me that walking was the one activity that my handicap had not curtailed, an activity that I could do, and one which gave me a great deal of pleasure. The idea was formed and began to take shape..... all that was needed was a little training, the distribution of a few sponsor forms, to get myself to one end or other of Britain - and then I could start walking!

I mentioned the idea to my wife, expecting perhaps a little cautious enthusiasm, and a degree of approbation for my public-spirited thinking. I couldn't have been more wrong. The overriding reaction to my idea was a combination of horror and ridicule.

We had been married for 45 years and I had thought there was little I could do to surprise her after so long, but she clearly considered that I had come up with the craziest of crazy schemes and that I should be persuaded to forget all about it as soon as possible. I was disappointed by her reaction, since I knew that I would need her full support, but in some ways, it only made me more determined to find a way to carry out my scheme, and to convince her that it could be done.

3

Perhaps other members of the family, and close friends would give my idea a more enthusiastic reception? Again I was disappointed. In general they refused to take it seriously and just laughed.

Those who realised that I really intended to go ahead tried to convince me of the impossibility of the scheme:

"How will you find your way?" I was asked-
"How will you find somewhere to stay along the route?"
"What if something goes wrong?"
"How will your wife and family cope with the worry ?"
"What if....?"

The questions went on, and to most of them I could give some sort of answer. The ones about ensuring my safety and causing anxiety to my family were more difficult. There had to be a way to do such a walk safely, and to minimise their concern.

I was taken aback by the fears of my friends and family. I have always been very independent, and I assumed that because I was sound of wind and limb and confident of being able to cope with a 900 mile walk from one end of Britain to the other, that others would share my confidence. Perhaps the fact that I was 65 years old, and registered as a blind person had something to do with their concern. I have some sight, and the little I have is quite good. I have a very small area (about the size of a pinhead) of central vision, often referred to as "tunnel vision". However, if the light conditions are bad, or I am suffering from one of the frequent headaches which result from trying to make the most of my residual eyesight, then even this area of vision deteriorates.

Eventually the opposition eased a little, and at last a constructive comment emerged. It was suggested that if someone else went with me who would be able to find overnight accommodation, guide me through the towns and difficult road junctions and to keep in regular telephone contact with my wife then the idea might become a possibility. This would enable my wife to know where I was, and to co-ordinate any help if it was needed.

This may seem a perfectly obvious solution, but I was not happy with it. This is because of the degree of concentration I need to employ when walking. I have to be constantly aware of the position of the kerb, white line or verge and any distraction can be disastrous. If I become disoriented, it is only by focusing on the precise spot that I need that I can get back in the right position. Sighted people see things, like the kerb, in relation to the things around them, like the road, and the grass or the pavement. I can only see what I am looking at, and imagine the vast area of road I need to examine, a pinhead at a time, before I can find the edge of it. The danger, of course, is that I can unwittingly drift out into the road and into the path of oncoming traffic.

Someone else walking with me, no matter how congenial their company, would make the necessary concentration impossible. Also, I wanted to travel at my own speed and stop or go according to my own needs. In my view, road walking with a companion was not on.

Nevertheless I was determined not to be put off, and eventually agreed that I would be content to have a vehicle and driver as a back up. If a team could be found to back me up for various stretches of the route, to go ahead and watch out for potential difficulties and arrange accommodation then I could count on the support of my wife. People began to realise that I was serious, and I was now in a position to start enlisting some real help and making detailed plans.

Having heard about the "Fight for Sight" Campaign organised by Moorfields Hospital in order to raise money for research into all types of blindness and eye disorders, not just R.P. I decided that I would make my walk part of this campaign. I knew some of the people involved in the "Fight for Sight" and was aware of the dedication, time and effort they put into their work. I wrote to the organisers of the campaign, explaining what I intended to do, and they agreed to send information, stickers, collecting tins and any items to help with fund raising. There was considerable interest in my plan, and I was asked for more details, such as when did I plan to go, and how long would it take ?

Suddenly an apparently impossible idea had become a reality. I was actually going to walk 900 miles to raise money for the research and treatment of blindness.

It was now almost Christmas and I had to time my walk for April or May in order to benefit from the maximum amount of daylight. I had to start planning with some urgency. I had to decide whether to walk from Land's End to John O'Groats or vice versa. I knew that if a driver and a vehicle were only available for a limited amount of time, then they would be most useful to me in the remote, less populated areas of Scotland and during the Northern part of my journey. I therefore decided to walk from North to South, and to set off from John O'Groats, which up to now had only been a name on a map, only known because it is the northernmost tip of the United Kingdom, and to walk until I reached Land's End.

I informed the "Fight for Sight" Campaign that my walk would take place in May 1991 and that it would probably take about six weeks. I calculated that I could walk 20–23 miles each day provided I set off early enough to finish in good daylight. Once the light begins to fail, the onset of dusk robs me of any sight and I am completely night-blind.

It was during January that the postman brought a small parcel of stickers and leaflets to our cottage on the Long Mynd. These would be used to publicise the purpose of the walk, and to help to raise money. My wife, Edna, sighed when she opened it, whether with resignation that the walk was really going to take place, or with anticipation that this was the beginning of a process that was to take over our lives for the next few months, I'm not sure.

The Preparation

At this point there were two main areas of preparation. One was the one that I could organise with confidence, and that was my own training schedule. I knew that I had to prepare myself for walking on main roads and teach myself the safest way to cross intersections and roundabouts. I also aimed to increase my walking speed from 3.5 mph to 4.0 mph without losing concentration on the edge of the road while cars and lorries were passing close to me.

The other matter was more difficult. We had tried to make a calculation about the costs of the undertaking and it would clearly be quite an expense. I listed the obvious things, and Edna wrote them down. I am told that my writing is so minute that it is very difficult to read although it looks alright to me... so Edna wrote;

*   Bed & Breakfast for two -40 nights at £15.00   £1200.00

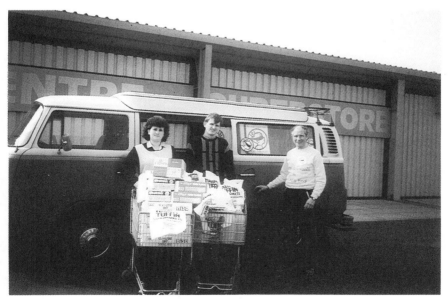

Preparation — Stocking up

• Food and provisions -£5 per person per day	£ 400.00
• Petrol for 2000 miles -£2 per gallon -40mpg	£ 100.00
• Walking boots and socks	£ 100.00
• Telephone and postage for fund-raising	£ 100.00
Total	£1900.00

As with all lists of prospective costs, I knew that there would be other expenses I hadn't thought of and that something would be needed as a reserve for emergencies. We did not include any allowance for vehicle hire or insurance, since we hoped that these might be donated along with the driver's services. It was clear that we had to find some way of getting some assistance with this funding. The organisers of the "Fight for Sight" charity suggested that I try to find a sponsor to meet some of these expenses. They offered to approach people on our behalf if we had any suggestions, and advised us that our best chance was to try local businesses.

The Training

I remained confident that all the difficulties would be overcome, and continued with my self-imposed training schedule. I was increasingly aware that no matter how hard my supporters worked, no matter how efficient the organisation, the actual carrying out of the task was my responsibility, and I had to be sure that I was in the best possible physical shape and prepared for all foreseeable eventualities.

I had no fear of walking long distances, since it was my main form of relaxation to walk for miles across the unpopulated Shropshire hills, but that was hill walking, on soft surfaces and without the threat of traffic. The task I had set myself provided a new set of challenges.

I did not know how well my feet and legs would stand up to long distances on hard surfaces and I discovered that after about thirteen miles of road walking the ball of my left foot became sore. This was the only difficulty I encountered and a cushioned pad under that part of my foot ensured that I had no further problems.

There were much greater problems, however, when it came to dealing with busy roads and heavy traffic. Like most people who enjoy walking as a form of relaxation, I avoided roads whenever possible and now I knew that I had to get used to them. I chose the A49 between Ludlow and Shrewsbury since it is a busy single carriageway with very little pavement or provision for pedestrians, and therefore typical of many of the roads I would be walking along on my journey.

The lack of pavement was in fact an advantage. It is easier to walk on the road, and there are fewer obstacles . The hazards littered along most pavements make walking a nightmare for anyone who is blind or partially sighted. There are ill-placed telegraph poles, litter bins and hydrants. There are irregular and uneven dips at each driveway, frequent roads to cross, and worst of all, parked cars blocking much of the path. No, I would be infinitely safer on the road!

At the start of my serious training, I realised that I had a natural tendency to stop and look when I heard a heavy vehicle coming towards me. I knew that I had to cure myself of this because, in the process of trying to make out the vehicle, I would step sideways into the road, terrifying myself, and the driver. By this time I would have lost the road edge, and it would take some time to rediscover it, especially since it

9

was rarely where I thought it ought to be.

I experimented with walking along both sides of the road. It soon became clear to me that there were two serious disadvantages to walking on the right. Firstly, the draught from oncoming large or high-sided vehicles would at times almost stop me, and secondly my back-up vehicle would find it more difficult to stay in contact, particularly on dual carriageways.

After a few days, I found that I became accustomed to the rumble and whine of traffic as it passed me, and this, together with the fact that I was often too busy concentrating on where I was going to think about anything else meant that I was soon able to ignore it altogether.

Looking back at the preparations

While I was busy preparing myself physically and mentally for the actual walk, a process which I controlled and which showed steady and tangible results, the other side of the whole operation proceeded less smoothly. There was lots of positive help, and I came across many wonderful and spontaneously generous people during this time. However, there were also disappointments and setbacks and at times an almost overwhelming array of administrative and organisational problems.

By now, Edna had become the chief administrator for the project. In spite of still having some reservations about the wisdom or sanity of the undertaking, her support and efforts were unconditional, and I could not have managed without her. The kitchen of our cottage, with its large, old scrubbed deal table became the centre of operations, and the pace of our quiet country days changed considerably.

Although the aim of my walk was to raise money, and fund-raising inevitably means publicity, I did not enjoy the thought of becoming in any way a public figure. For this reason, I really appreciated the sympathetic and helpful approach from our local newspaper, The Shropshire Star and from John King, of Radio Shropshire.

The Shropshire Star accompanied their informative article with a photograph, one of the few in existence which really looks like me and we were able to reproduce this and incorporate it into the official sponsor forms so that people would understand who I was and what I was doing.

In the Radio Shropshire interview, I was able to explain that I was looking for support drivers, and this resulted in an offer from a man called Eric Richardson to accompany me for one week. He explained that he would very much like to help, but that he could only do so during April as he was going on holiday early in May.

Two other offers followed; Harry Field, a fellow member of our local walking group, the Bishop's Castle Footpath Group, offered to take me to John O'Groats for the start of the walk and accompany me as far as Edinburgh. It was most convenient for him to do his stint at Easter, and since Easter Sunday was the first of April it seemed a particularly appropriate date to begin. I was very relieved by Harry's generous offer of help, for this first part of the journey was the one that I was most concerned about, and I knew that I would need adequate support. Then came another offer from a friend of long-standing, Wilf Barnett. He was prepared to take over from Harry, and travel with me for one week from Edinburgh.

At this stage everything seemed to be going well. I had a driver to take me to the start, and to accompany me for the first week. I had drivers for the two following weeks, by which time I hoped to be as far on my journey as Hereford, not far from my own home, and I felt sure that the rest of the journey would present few problems.

The search for a vehicle proved to be a greater problem than the search for drivers. The "Fight for Sight" organisers had approached Rover Cars Ltd. on my behalf, since I had worked for them or their predecessors over a forty year period. They expressed a willingness to help, and did offer the loan of a car but since this could only be for very short periods of one or two days I had to keep up the search.

When I first started work, at the age of 14, it had been at the Drew's Lane plant of British Leyland (later Leyland Daf Ltd.) I was working there when it was bombed, and returned to work there after some years in the Royal Air Force. I remember the first production of the Morris Minor, and felt very involved with the history of motor vehicle manufacture in the Midlands. I approached Leyland Daf. Ltd. explaining some of this background, and explaining what I needed. The initial response was very encouraging; if I arranged comprehensive insurance, made sure that all drivers were experienced, and contributed an article to their Company magazine then they would loan us a vehicle. I went ahead with the arrangements feeling very relieved that the problem had been solved.

Countdown to take off

Day One minus nine

We were informed that Leyland Daf Ltd. did not have a vehicle available for us. I spoke to my son, Frank, who is a G.P. in practice in the West Midlands. he has a wide circle of friends and acquaintances, and I knew that if anyone could help us at this stage, it would be him.

He had a friend who was going to new Zealand for six weeks, and was prepared to lend us his Volkswagen Caravanette. He warned us that it was twelve years old and of doubtful reliability, but it sounded like the answer to a prayer. A caravanette would also provide emergency accommodation if it became necessary, and so I was grateful to accept this offer.

Day One minus eight

Edna drove Harry and I the 25 miles to Telford to collect the Caravanette. It looked fine if a little battered and our spirits rose. An hour later, we were still trying to start it. Our combined efforts were proving fruitless, maybe because Edna and Harry had little mechanical experience and I could see very little. A very, very nice man from the A.A. came to our rescue and it took him only a few minutes to persuade the engine to turn. He advised us to get the van checked over thoroughly before embarking on our journey. Appreciating the wisdom of this advice, we arranged with a local garage to check it for us, and to let us know if there was any major defect to be put right, or large expense to be met in order to make it roadworthy. It was not until much later that we discovered that this instruction had been interpreted to mean that if it would start up each day, there was no problem.

Day One minus seven

Many sponsor forms had gone out, and enough donations had come in for us to open a special bank account.

Our local Supermarket, Harry Tuffin's at Craven Arms offered some supplies. We would be presented with £130.00 of basic foods by Roy Delves, the generous proprietor, who had carefully selected items which would be most useful.

I needed to insure the vehicle, and I approached Legal and General Insurance. I explained why I wanted the insurance, and what I was doing. The response was immediate and more generous than I could have dreamed. Not only did they offer us free insurance for the vehicle, but asked what walking boots I would be wearing, and when I explained that I had just bought a pair of Brasher boots for £70.00, they paid for those as well. Thus armed with their good wishes, and two large, colourful umbrellas we felt that things were really going well.

Day One minus six

Time to review the situation.

We had received many offers of accommodation along the route, but some were only available on certain dates and it was difficult trying to sort out which ones we would be able to use.

I was spending some part of every day out walking. I was also trying to visit as many businesses as I could in person in order to raise funds. This was very time consuming, but also very rewarding, not only for the money and promises of money, but for the interest shown and the people I met.

It was surprising how many people I spoke to either suffered from or had been treated for some serious eye problem, and everyone seemed to know someone who was losing their sight through some disorder or other, so a rebuff was rare and most of the money promised on these occasions came into the fund.

I always explained on such visits that all the money donated would go directly to the "Fight for Sight" and that I was financing the trip myself. I hoped that perhaps one or two understanding companies might be able to assist me with the expenses of the walk but I soon realised that many of them were struggling through the recession and had little to spare. I was able to understand this, and although there were few corporate donations, the people I spoke to generally made a generous personal contribution for which I was most grateful.

Day One minus five

I come from a large, warm-hearted family, and I was not surprised to find that some of them wanted to do more to help than just make a contribution. I should say at this point that there were several offers of help from both family and friends that for one reason or another, I was not able to take up. I would like to say that these offers, although they never became translated into practical help, formed part of the tide of goodwill which kept me going, and helped me to overcome every difficulty along the way.

Two of my brothers-in-law offered to take over the support driving for the final part of the journey, and were prepared to use their own vehicles. This was very good news, not least because it took some of the pressure off Edna who was snowed under with providing information, sorting out sponsor forms, answering queries, not to mention organising food and clothing and vehicle change-overs. We now had drivers for the whole journey, and we knew that the first change would take place after one week, in Edinburgh. We had to make a calculated guess about where we would be for the following changes of driver.

Day One minus four

My training was now almost complete.

I was able to walk confidently along A roads and ignore the traffic. I was sure that I could safely cross islands and deal with intersections although there may me many people who are still bemused at catching sight of an elderly man with a white cane constantly crossing and re-crossing a road by listening for gaps in the traffic.

I had also succeeded in increasing my walking speed. For this I had enlisted the aid of a friend who is a marathon runner, and a naturally fast walker. He stayed with us for a while and I trailed after him for many miles. Sometimes I had to trot to keep up with him but gradually this became less and less necessary, and I knew that I was now walking at the speed I wanted.

This part of the training was carried out among the south Shropshire hills and many times we found ourselves in ditches or walking into posts or tree stumps and rolling ignominiously down a hillside. We got lost several times, and on one occasion when we asked a farmer for directions and explained that we could not see the landmarks he was talking about, he just pointed us in the right direction and offered his sympathy by saying;

"You don't make one good 'un between the pair of you"

My companion on these unusual hillside hikes was David Winsper, who like me is a registered blind person. He has a small amount of peripheral vision and a little night sight but no colour vision. Since I can see colours but am completely night blind, and my remaining vision is central... the farmers observation was very close to the truth!

David is someone who, like me ,was able to laugh while crawling out of a muddy bog which lay unseen on our route, and regards bruised shins and unexpected tumbles as a small price to pay for the pleasure of independence and freedom. David's record of achievements includes several marathons, including three London ones, and he has travelled from Land's End to John O'Groats on the back of a tandem. More recently, he has obtained the distinction of being the first blind man to complete the Long Mynd Hike. This is a gruelling 50 mile cross country walk which involves about 8.000 feet of climbing. All this is done carrying full survival kit and takes place during October, when much of the walking has to be done in the dark. I was disappointed on that occasion to have to give up after 22 miles with a damaged knee, and with increased admiration for David whose determination is a real inspiration.

Thanks to my training companion, then, I was now feeling more than ready to begin my own marathon walk.

Day One minus three

Harry collected the caravanette from the garage and brought it to the cottage so that we could pack and complete our preparations. It started up on the first attempt and ran reasonably smoothly and all seemed to be well. Harry was concerned about a leak where water had dripped into the van near to the sink. He had some experience of similar vehicles, and was worried that in wet weather it could become very uncomfortable. I was prepared to be philosophical about it, especially since we did not have much choice!

The caravanette looked a whole lot better after it had been thoroughly cleaned and the loose number plate fixed. The sun was shining and I was not put off even by the fact that the bolt securing the spare wheel was rusted so solid that it had to be sawn off and replaced. I was now growing impatient to be on my way.

Day One minus two

Harry and I, accompanied by Edna drove to Harry Tuffin's Supermarket, where we were presented with their donation of supplies.

It was now important to ensure that everything we needed was packed into the caravanette. We had a full bottle of gas for the cooker and heater, and we had been loaned a new, fully charged heavy duty battery so that the light would not be a drain on the vehicle battery. We had warm sleeping bags. All that remained was to pack a bag with personal clothing and necessities. Again I had one of Edna's invaluable lists to help;

1. Socks (seamless) cotton
2. Socks (seamless) woollen . For wearing over cotton socks.
3. Waterproof coat with hood. Bright yellow
4. Waterproof leggings. Bright Yellow
5. Woollen hat and gloves
6. Tracksuit
7. Training shoes
8. Sweatshirts. Bright colours. Printed "John O'Groats to Land's End
9. Boots . 3 pairs New Brasher boots
   Recently acquired Hawkins boots
   Old, repaired ,comfortable boots.
10. Rucksack
11. Spare shirts and trousers
12. Underwear.
13. Warm Arran sweater.

I intended to wear a bum bag for small personal items, and of course I would have to carry my white cane. For the first time, it seemed to me, the cane was not a symbol of a disability that I resented, but a symbol of what I was trying to do and an expression of my determination to succeed.

All these items fitted easily into my one zipped bag, and I was a little taken aback when I realised that Harry seemed to have packed at least a dozen bags with his personal effects... perhaps I counted some of them twice!

All the bags went into the van. We added a first-aid kit, well stocked with plasters provided by well-wishers anticipating a few blisters.

By the time we had packed everything, and added some collecting tins in case we had any opportunity for fund-raising while the walk was in progress, there was scarcely room for me in the van. At last all was ready. Edna had prepared a notebook for Harry in which he had details of people to telephone, to send postcards to and directions for finding the flat in Edinburgh where we were to stay. There was money for petrol and other expenses and a specially drawn up sheet of paper which would be completed each day as a log of my progress and signed by someone at each place.

The plan was to set off early the next morning, to travel most of the day and after an overnight stop go on to John O'Groats to begin the walk.

If I had had any thoughts about a quiet, restful evening before the start of the journey North, then it was soon dispelled by the arrival of my son and daughter with their respective families. Five excited grandchildren aged from 5 to 13 wanted to know everything about what I was going to do. They had made large scale maps of Britain, and intended to trace my progress along each part of the route. They had no doubt that I would achieve my aim, and their confidence was at once heartening and yet quite a responsibility. I could not let them down.

Day One minus one - The journey North

Despite the overcrowded, noisy house and the impossibility of an early night, I was up by 6 O'clock and after a shower and a good breakfast, was anxious to be off. Harry arrived punctually just before 7 O'clock and we were ready to go.

My home village, which scarcely merits the name, consists of three or four farms, some very ancient dwellings inhabited by folk whose lifestyle has changed little in the last fifty years, and who have only recently decided on the innovation of an indoor toilet, and two or three "newcomers" like me, who have adapted or converted the old weather-beaten country properties into more convenient homes. My newness has worn off a little after 25 years. A much more recent arrival, Pete Postlethwaite , was there to give me a send off, in spite of the early hour. Pete is a colourful character, who is rapidly making a name for himself as a talented actor. He had given me a lot of support , not only by inflicting sponsor forms on the entire cast of the play he was appearing in in London, but also by loaning invaluable detailed maps of much of Scotland and arranging for me to stay with his brother-in-law in Edinburgh at that stage of the journey.

On a cold, bright morning, the 30th March, the tiny village was quiet except for the knot of people around our cottage gate. It was a hopeful start, and with encouraging smiles and waves from family and neighbours, we set off.

Bouyed up by good wishes, and scarcely believing that I was actually on my way, I felt that nothing now could stop me from reaching my goal. I paid little attention to Harry's trepidation about the state of the caravanette, and felt convinced that it would keep going somehow.

Harry drove carefully, clearly anxious not to overstrain the vehicle. The first part of the journey was comfortable, if a little noisy and we both began to relax. I tried to pick up some details about the road we were travelling along, the A49, knowing that if all went well, I would be walking down this same stretch of road in a few weeks time.

Our peace of mind was shattered when, ninety minutes into the journey, an ominous loud clanging and clumping announced the collapse of the exhaust pipe. It was clearly unrepairable, so we pulled it off, and for some unknown reason, we carefully stowed this foot or so of rusty, useless metal inside the caravanette.

Having decided that nothing could be done about it, we continued on our way. There was no significant difference, except perhaps it was a little noisier, but the incident had disturbed Harry and increased his nervousness about the reliability of the vehicle.

The remainder of the journey through England continued uneventfully and pleasantly. We stopped for lunch near Penrith and again there was a hint of trouble to come when the motor showed some reluctance to start up again after the break. Nevertheless things continued to run smoothly and indeed by the time we had skirted Glasgow and reached Perth, the caravenette was rattling along and seemed to be going better as we went on. Although it was getting dark by this time, and beginning to drizzle, Harry decided that he would keep going until we reached Inverness, so that there would be an easy day's run left for the next day. I was happy with this and we were both feeling very satisfied with the day's progress when we stopped at a small roadside restaurant about twelve miles from Inverness for a cup of tea and to fill up with fuel. It seemed to be an excellent opportunity to make sure that the caravanette was all ready for the following day, since we anticipated that there might not be too many petrol stations open on a Sunday.

This welcoming roadside cafe was at a place called Tomatin.

Replete with fuel, the vehicle refused to start. Not to be beaten, we left it for a few minutes while we went for a cup of tea, aware that a cup of tea can work wonders. This time there was no miracle, the tired old motor had had enough, and the battery was getting flatter with each attempt to start up.

The end of the beginning

Eventually even the best efforts of the nicest possible man from the AA failed to evoke a response from the worn out engine, and it seemed that we were stranded, transportless. It was a dark and cheerless night. Nights are always dark for me, but this one was dark for everyone. It was cold and drizzling and Harry seemed to be totally demoralised. He suggested that we should bow to the inevitable, find our way back home somehow and perhaps try again another time.

I could not accept defeat so easily. I thought of the effort that had gone into getting us this far, and was tempted to pack my rucksack and continue making my way northwards, no matter how slow and difficult it might prove to be. Harry and I were wrapped in our separate misery when the AA man returned from helping a couple whose motorbike had broken down. His much more positive attitude was just what we needed. He suggested that he

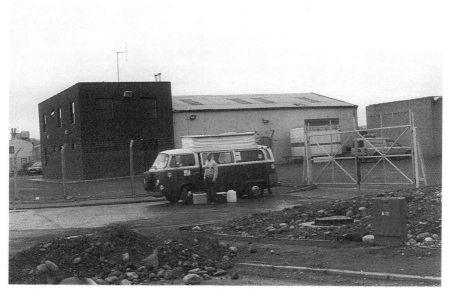

Break Down

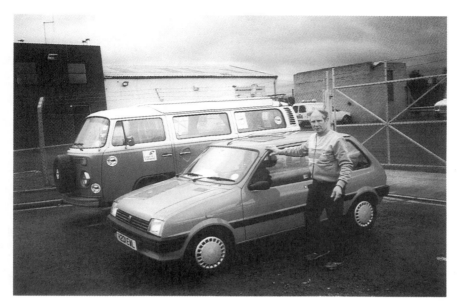

Hire Car

tow us into Inverness, where we could get a good night's sleep and then consider our situation in the morning.

Somehow we found the energy to get the caravanette in position for the tow. When we had moved it from the fuel pumps we had pushed it down a slope into a corner, and it was a heavy and awkward vehicle to manhandle in the dark on a wet slippery surface. It took an hour of struggling and pushing to get it lined up, and at this point, with morale at an all time low, we set off on a twelve mile hair raising journey behind the AA van. Harry had never been towed before and didn't like not being in control of the vehicle.

Our speed never rose above 25 mph but my impression gained from a perception of headlights coming towards us from the opposite side of the road and from Harry's tension was that we were speeding along at over 100mph and out of control. It was a terrifying experience.

When we reached Inverness we were cold, tired and more than a little damp round the edges. We parked the Caravanette in a quiet spot near to the AA compound. Aware of our difficulties, the AA man, whose name is Graham Scott, did all he could to help. He offered us the use of the AA facilities to telephone home to assure our supporters that we were O.K. It was too late to offer detailed explanations, and the effort needed to sound

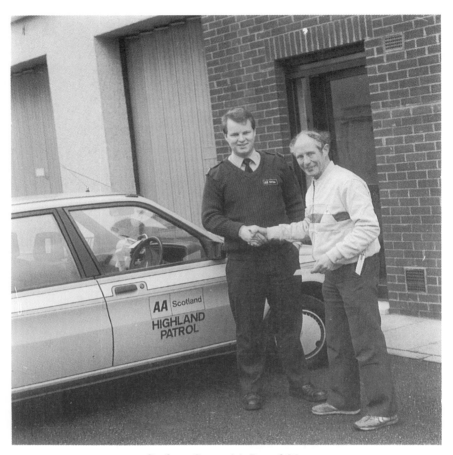

Graham Scott. AA Patrol Man

positive and hopeful was too great. I just told Edna that we had broken down and offered the idea that Harry had mooted of hiring a car in order to continue with our plans. We then were able to get washed, and while we drank a coffee Graham had made for us, we began to feel a little more human, and were able to consider in more detail the real possibility of hiring transport.

I really feel that without the cheerful presence and willing help of Graham Scott, this could have spelt the end of our enterprise. We were wet, cold, tired and unable to think straight, and his support undoubtedly set us back on road in more than one sense. Thank you Graham, your part was not a small one in this story.

Two decisions were made before Harry and I returned to the caravanette for a quick supper of hot soup and collapsed into our beds. These were that we should arrange for the caravanette to be sent back to my son's house as I knew I could rely on him to deal with it appropriately, and secondly that we should hire a car, preferably a Rover Metro, with which Harry was familiar. He said that it would be economical to run, easy to park, and roomy enough for the two of us and our pared down luggage. We would then need to find bed and breakfast accommodation at each stopping place along the way. Graham offered help to carry out our decisions, and offered to return in the morning.

Day One

It was a bright, cold morning. Our exhausted sleep had refreshed us and we indulged in a huge cooked breakfast washed down with several cups of tea. This set us up well for the day to come and ensured that we could face anything. We discussed which items of luggage we could take with us and how we should pack it in the limited space of a car boot o that we could have easy and swift access to items needed along the route. Everything else would have to go back with the caravanette.

Promptly at nine, Graham arrived and he and Harry sorted out the appropriate documents and set off to hire a car. This left me to continue sorting out what would be wanted on the journey. My personal clothing and possessions were packed in to a holdall, for spare clothes and a rucksack for waterproofs, torch, talking alarm clock, tea-maker and toiletries. These two bags, plus a bum bag and boots were to remain with me for the whole of the journey, and it was particularly important that I packed them myself, and kept them in order. If things are not where I expect them to be, I have difficulty locating them and it is enormously frustrating to spend time searching for something, when you know it is somewhere under your nose!

I also ensured that there was a good supply of cold drink in various flavours to go in the boot of the car.

It was a different Harry that returned a little later. A relieved grin had replaced the anxious frown, and only then did I realise what a strain it had been for him driving an unknown and unreliable vehicle for such a distance, and how seriously he was taking the responsibility for my success. I owe much to Harry's determination and bravery, not to mention staying power in the face of adversity.

Harry, with Graham's assistance, had hired a Rover Metro, which with the rear seat laid flat, gave us an adequate luggage area. We packed spare clothes, collecting tins and other things first, so that the drinks and provisions we would need en route were easily accessible. There was another advantage here in the design of the car, for in wet weather, the raised boot lid provided a nominal shelter for those times when I took a quick snack to keep up my energy. It was considered essential by both of us to keep the small gas bottle and burner, kettle, water and good supply of tea-bags close to hand. What great enterprise could go ahead without sufficient supplies of tea?

At last we were ready and anxious to be on our way on the last leg of our outward journey to John O'Groats.

Before we parted from Graham, he wished us luck and made a generous donation to the Fight For Sight. He also made sure we had good directions for finding our way on to the A9. I discovered later that Graham had also persuaded the hire car agent to organise the hire before he came for Harry at nine a.m. - and all this on Easter Sunday, after he had been with us until nearly midnight on the previous day ,which was his rest day! I am sure that the AA cannot take all the credit for the enormous generosity of Graham's personality, for he is indeed an extraordinary ' very, very nice man'.

We were on our way again, a little light-headed after all that had gone before, and in high spirits. Harry was relaxed and positive, and I was keen to start walking. I had already conceived the idea of starting out straight away and as we passed through Tore, Ardullie and Alness, I was trying to pick out and store any useful information about bypasses, bridges or junctions.

I think Harry thought I was mad when I told him that I wanted to start walking that day and that I would try to reach Wick. I suggested that we should look for bed and breakfast accommodation in Wick as we passed through. It was rather ambitious, and perhaps I should have given myself a bit more time to recover from the ordeal of the previous evening, but Harry could see that I was anxious to get started and agreed to my plan, adding that he could always pick me up before I reached Wick if I grew too tired and take me the rest of the way by car. There was something a bit absurd in this idea, since I would then have to be taken back the next morning to the point where I had stopped...but there was much that was absurd about this whole scheme .

We travelled on, passed Alness and along the A836, through the Struie Pass and on to Bonar Bridge. We followed the coast road, bypassing Dornoch where we could see that a new bridge was under construction across Dornoch Firth. We now turned once again onto the A9, this was the road that went all the way to John O'Groats.

It was strange, this last stage of the journey. We were travelling quite fast, but my impatience made it seem interminable. It felt to me as if we had been on the road for days and yet it was only yesterday that we had set off from our Shropshire home. The fact that we had got this far was in some measure due to the fact that I refused to entertain any doubts about achieving what I had set out to do. Maybe my tunnel vision worked on more than one level, but with hindsight I am aware of just how much of the peripheral responsibilities were shouldered by my supporters and in particular, at this stage, by Harry.

Through Golspie, Brora, Helmsdale and on to Wick. Names that were fixed in my mind after long hours spent studying the map and piecing together a picture of the route I must follow.

The first house in Wick had a B & B sign. It was the most southerly house in the town and therefore easy for me to find. Harry reported it to be clean and pleasant, and had reserved us a room for that night. At last things seemed to be going our way, and off we went again on the final 17 miles to John O'Groats.

It was twenty minutes before two p.m. when Harry parked the car. There was time for a sandwich lunch, a cup of coffee and a bar of chocolate before I visited the Hotel where the manager went through the ritual of signing and dating our form and enquired how we intended to make the journey. He must have had many strange answers to that standard enquiry and expressed no surprise when he discovered that I was blind !

It only remained for Harry and I to take a commemorative photograph of each other on the START line, to take a cursory look at John O'Groats since we were there, and to decide that it was not worth fund raising amongst the two or three coach loads of damp tourists who looked much more interested in returning to their warm hotels, a final fuelling cup of tea and then, at a quarter past two. I set out.

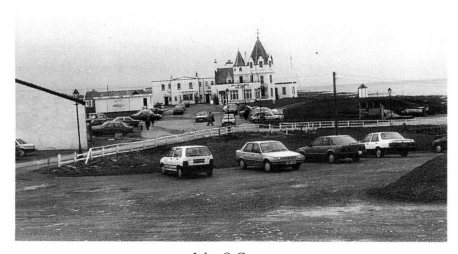

John-O-Groats

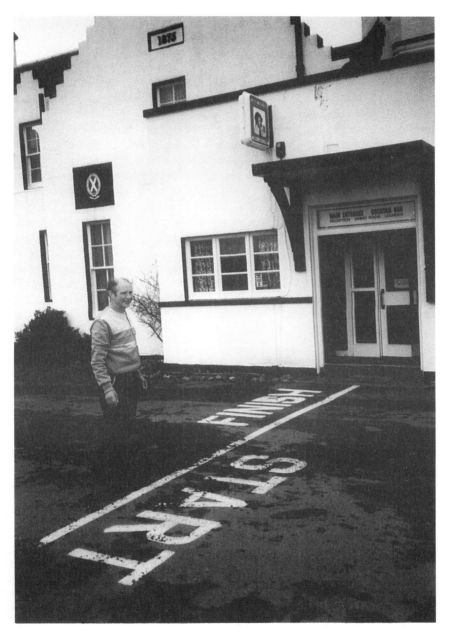

The Start Line

27

It was not a momentous moment, a shortish, balding grandfather setting out for a walk, carrying a white cane to indicate his disability, and wearing a warm woolly hat and bright yellow waterproof leggings and jacket against the persistent drizzle. In spite of that, it felt very good to be on my way at last, and I was determined to reach Wick before 7 o'clock that evening.

Kreiss, Reiss and on to Wick. The words gave a rhythm to my steps and it was a hopeful start.

After an hour the drizzle eased and although it was bitterly cold, my legs were uncomfortably hot in the waterproof leggings and I decided to take them off. This was no simple undertaking when wearing boots. I managed to get the leggings down as far as my knees and then I needed to stand on one leg in an attempt to ease the hem of the leggings over my other boot. Naturally I soon overbalanced and tried to hop in order to stay upright. However, since I began this manoeuvre on a quite a gradient, the hopping became faster and faster until I finished in a heap at the bottom of the hill.

I realised that my performance had had an audience when two men peered down at me, and scarcely hiding their laughter asked me if I was alright and made sure that I wasn't hurt. Apart from a muddy arm, and a wet seat and perhaps a little dented dignity, there was no harm done. The Scottish gentlemen, who had been pushing their bicycles up the hill, searched their pockets for a donation when they discovered what I was doing, and apologised for the limited funds this search produced, saying that a stunt like that was worth at least a pound. They continued on their way, still chuckling. I eventually managed to divest myself of the troublesome leggings, only to find that the dry spell was to be a brief one and that the persistent drizzle was to be my companion for the rest of the way.

When I met up with Harry, I was able to put the waterproof leggings back on in relative comfort, sitting in the car, but by this time, my trousers and legs were damp. The subsequent discomfort taught me to wear leggings whenever it was wet, and to keep them on until I was sure that the rain was over. The inconvenience of walking in leggings was far outweighed by the discomfort of walking in wet clothes.

Harry had, meanwhile, been working out the best method of using the car as a support for me. It was obviously impractical to drive at walking pace, and he experimented with driving from lay-by to lay-by. This scheme was not very satisfactory as there were either several lay-bys clustered together, or none for long distances. I suggested that he drive on for about four miles, and we meet up at approximately hourly intervals. Harry thought this was too risky this early in the walk and we came up with the compromise that he should wait while I walked for fifteen minutes, then drive for two miles and wait. This way we were never more than one mile, or fifteen minutes walk apart.

There were occasions when this arrangement was not possible, but generally the system worked well and we used it until we reached Edinburgh. My other drivers had their own ideas, but we will come to those later.

I have been told that the coastline that I walked along on this first afternoon is rugged and picturesque and a complete contrast to the dull, treeless, featureless moorland of the inland scenery. I can give no personal impression of the beauty of my surroundings since the poor light and the constant drizzle ensured that I could see nothing of them.

I should perhaps explain that if some of my descriptions seem a little strange, it is because I can only describe how things are to me, and that is not always as they appear to other people. I remember once describing a beautiful unspoilt area that I had walked through when my listener wondered what had happened to the cement works that was situated in that spot. I can only presume that nothing had happened to the cement works, but that my own peculiar view of things had kindly obliterated it from the scene.

Harry was very watchful on that first afternoon, he would look for my approach, and make sure that I had a drink if I needed one and check that all was well before I continued on.

I reached one meeting point before Harry expected me. He had not begun to look out for me, and I simply did not see the parked car as I walked by. I passed within a few feet of him without either of us knowing! It did not occur to me that anything was amiss, but Harry, after waiting for ten minutes after the time he had expected me to appear, became very concerned and returned to the last place where he had seen me. He thought something terrible must have happened, and grew more and more bewildered at finding no sign of me. He did not know what to do, not believing that I could pass by without either of us knowing. Eventually he drove on, and it must have been a great relief to him when he finally caught up with me, for by this time I had covered quite a distance and was well on the way to Wick.

We arrived at our lodgings in Wick twenty minutes before the 7 O'clock deadline I had set myself, so the speed was right, and I was not unduly tired. However, I was hungry and eager to get out of my damp clothes and cleaned up so that we could go out to eat.

Mrs. Bremner, the landlady, had recommended a place for a good meal. But first, a shower. I entered the shower hopefully, switched it on, and gasped as a jet of icy water hit me. I fumbled around and found another switch and a tap, but could make out no symbols. I tried every combination of switches but all I could achieve was a variation in the force and flow, but no variation in the temperature of the water. Shivering, I dried myself as quickly as possible and returned to the bedroom. Harry went off for a shower, and I waited for his reaction...when he returned it was obvious that he had found the secret to warm water. I had the dubious satisfaction of remembering that someone once told me that cold showers are good for you!

It was time for me to report back to Edna. At last, a more positive and cheerful telephone call. Mrs. Bremner was happy for me to use the telephone, and I gave Edna my number to call me back so that I could talk with an easy conscience. I was aware of the mounting cost of the hire car, and suggested that it might be worth another attempt to enlist the support of Rover. It was good to report that the first stage of the walk had been completed, and easy to think that from now one it would all go according to plan.

We had an excellent meal at a Restaurant about half a mile away. It was run by two young women who supplied soup, chicken fillet and vegetables, apple pie , cakes, and a pot of tea before and after the meal, and feeling pleasantly full and relaxed, we strolled back afterwards. The rain had stopped and the wind had eased.

I studied the map for a little while, memorising place names and any unusual features and went to bed at about ten p.m. Harry was by this time relaxing in front of the television. A satisfactory end to day one.

Day Two

I was eager to get an early start for the first full day of walking, hoping to set a pattern from the outset. I had arranged breakfast for half past seven, as this was the earliest I could reasonably ask for it. A large appetising breakfast was ready for me and in addition Mrs. Bremner had prepared for us a generous packed lunch and filled our flask with coffee for no extra charge. Thanks to her kindness and support it was easy to put our previous difficulties behind us and feel that at last things were going well.

I had been thinking about Harry, and trying to think of a way that he could take a short break from his painstaking job of taking responsibility for my safety and well being. I realised that the days must seem very long to him, for while I was striding out, he was spending much of his time waiting and watching for me. He was reading a great deal, and I think he must have reached a very interesting part of his book when I walked past him on the previous day! I managed to persuade him that I was confident about my route for that day, and that he need not worry about catching up with me for a couple of hours. This giving him a breathing space, chance to do a little

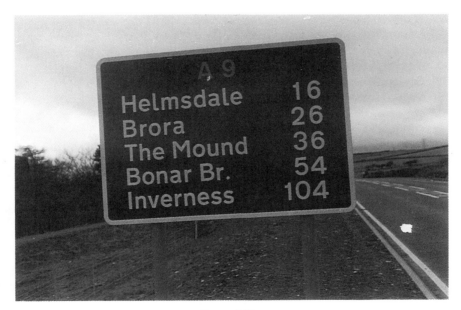

Second Day

31

shopping, and also the opportunity to buy postcards of the area, and ensure that the log keeping track of my progress was signed and dated.

At eight o'clock I set out. The wind hit me as I stepped out of the door. It was directly in my face, but rather than being dismayed by this, my feeling of well being was such that I positively enjoyed the thought of the extra challenge of walking against the wind. At least it wasn't raining and I didn't need to wear cumbersome waterproofs.

I also revelled in the thought that I could push on for two hours at my own pace, and get as far along the road as possible without a 'minder', just as every child perceives that caring parents restrict their freedom, and love to steal a little independence, prepared to take any risks involved. I felt a pleasure in my solitude and hoped that Harry, in spite of his solicitous care, would be able to do the same.

I began to grow concerned that the strong headwind was slowing down my pace. I had asked Harry to record the exact mileage for me so that when we met up I would know exactly how fast I was going. This stretch of the road follows the coast and when I dared to look I could see the grey, white-capped sea smashing into the rocks. Although this part of the road is fairly level, the force of the wind made it feel as though I were walking up hill all the time. My self-imposed schedule made it very important to keep up a steady speed and was beginning to think that it was impossible for me to maintain it in these conditions.

I was immensely pleased when I met up with Harry after two and a quarter hours and he informed me that I had walked nine miles. I was keeping up my pace. This seemed amazing to me, and I can only assume that having trained myself to walk at a particular speed, I had conditioned myself to put in the additional effort to maintain it even in adverse conditions.

I had walked through Ubster, Bruan and Clyth and on to Lybster. While I was going through Lybster, I came alongside a young woman with a child in a pushchair. I realised with a shock that she was the first pedestrian I had seen and by this time I was thirty miles from John'O Groats. I had been aware of traffic on the roads, and a few passing cyclists, but if there had been any pedestrians, even in Wick, then I had failed to notice them. It is fortunate that I had not entertained hopes of doing much spontaneous collecting of donations along this part of the route !

The young mother in Lybster, however, when she saw me, asked what I was doing the walk for. When she found out that I was raising funds for the 'Fight for Sight' she wished us luck and made a donation, remarking that her own mother was losing her sight. She also very kindly offered to make us some tea, but I had to refuse explaining that I was aiming to get to Helmsdale that day and that there wasn't time to stop. Since it was a further twenty three miles, my friendly informant was doubtful that I would in fact reach Helmsdale, but in the event that we did, she gave us the name of La Mirage Cafe, which she said was very comfortable and the food very good. I left her with some regrets about the cup of tea, but not for long, for soon after I became increasingly aware of the lack of roadside conveniences in that part of the country.

I grew more and more uncomfortable as I searched the bleak and open countryside for a ditch or hedge to offer some measure of privacy. Eventually I decided to use the ostrich approach...if I can't see you then you can't see me.

Shortly after this it began to rain hard. The driving rain in my face made it difficult to see with my head up so I had to bow my head and concentrate my vision on a point a yard or two in front of me. This reduced the amount I could see and it meant that I frequently stepped into puddles that I was unaware of until I felt the water running in over the top of my boots. By half past twelve when I stopped for lunch, my feet were soaked and I was glad of the opportunity to put on dry socks and boots.

With dry feet, and full of Mrs. Bremners excellent sandwiches, I was off again. Changing my footwear had been a mistake, because within a few minutes of setting out, my feet were as wet as ever. They did not feel cold or uncomfortable, though, so when an hour or so later the rain stopped, I dispensed with the waterproofs but did nothing about my feet. I felt better without the waterproofs, since the wind had been billowing them out so that I resembled the Michelin man. I pressed on through Latheron, Dumbeath and Berridale. At Berridale I suggested to Harry that it might be a good idea if he went on to Helmsdale to find a place where we could sleep that night . He agreed, and half an hour later when we met up, he said that he had booked us in at La Mirage. He suggested that as I had walked thirty miles and it was nearly five o'clock I should finish walking for the day at that point. I was tempted to walk the six miles into Helmsdale since the rain had stopped, but the promise of a hot bath and a change of clothes was more than I could resist so a quarter past five that evening saw us at La Mirage in Helmsdale.

La Mirage stands out among the sombre grey stone buildings of the village of Helmsdale, with its pink paint, and shiny prettily curtained windows. When I first saw such a a brightly feminine building in amongst its darkly respectable neighbours, I wondered exactly what Harry had arranged for us....perhaps this could explain why he had been so eager for me to finish my walk in good time!

Inside it is clean and bright with attractive coloured tablecloths and a profusion of flowers and pot pourris reminiscent of French hospitality. The

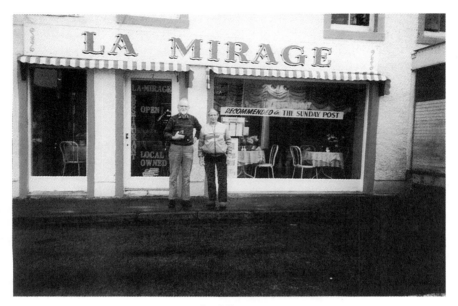

La Mirage

owner was indeed an attractive and attentive Scotswoman, but to my relief she showed no more than a landlady's interest in our well-being as she showed us our room and told us we could have a meal whenever we were ready. First, though, I wanted that bath.

This time there was no problem with the water temperature, it was lovely and warm. I put on dry clothes, and put the wet ones over radiators to dry. I stuffed my boots with paper and put them as near as possible to the warm radiators to dry as best they could. Next I went out to find a telephone to make my report home. Edna was surprised when I told her where we were. She had been watching the weather reports and knew that it was rough and was expecting us to report a delay. She also pointed out that there was no improvement forecast for the next day. Since it was a Bank Holiday, she had made no progress with attempts to get a replacement car, and the caravanette had not yet found its way back. I think she was relieved to hear that we had done so well and that apart from the wet and windy weather, all was going according to plan.

Duties done, Harry and I were now free to relax for the evening so we strolled back to La Mirage, ordered a meal, and over the essential pot of tea, discussed the day's progress and our future strategy. So far we had covered forty seven miles which was two days walk in our original plan so we had, at this point, gained a day. The fact that I was not tired surprised me and amazed Harry, who had been astonished to watch me running the last two hundred yards of my day's walk. This is something I do to relax my muscles. There is probably no rational explanation behind this practise, but it seems to work for me.

I surmised that if I had managed to walk thirty miles in the conditions of that Easter Monday, it was reasonable to think of thirty miles as an average day's target. It was not simply that I was in a hurry to cover the miles, but there was another consideration in the back of my mind now that the caravanette was out of action. This was the rapidly mounting cost of each day, which, with the car hire charges and accommodation for two would come to about £60. Thus being able to complete the walk in fewer days would represent a considerable amount off our total expenses.

After an excellent meal and delicious sweet we enjoyed a leisurely cup of coffee, then we retired, me to study my route, Harry to his book. My target for the following day was going to be Dornoch, another thirty miles on. I placed a straight edge on my large scale map, and with my finger moving slowly down , I memorised the names of the places I would pass through and any features of the landscape or deviations of the road that might be helpful for me to know. Breakfast was at eight in the morning, and this would mean a later start for me, and consequently a later finish which was not ideal. However, for the moment it was time for a good night's sleep.

Day Three

Tuesday the 2nd of April dawned sunny but still very windy. I was up just after six and spent some time sorting out clothes. Fortunately the damp things that had been put over radiators had all dried. My boots were still damp inside, but not too bad. During this investigation of the state of my gear, I was attempting to make as little noise as possible and allow Harry to sleep on undisturbed. The more I tried to be careful, the more I seemed to trip over unseen obstacles until it must have seemed to Harry as if a whole troop of intruders were crashing around the room. He got up at about seven, and we used the remaining time before breakfast to pack our things, and to stroll around the village and take a few photographs. I was growing restless and eager to be on the way.

Breakfast was cooked and served by the hostesses' son and was an excellent meal to which I scarcely did justice. Once again when we were due to set off we met with unsolicited generosity, for after filling our flask with coffee, we were presented with a bill which was only half of the full amount. This was another heartening example of the kindness we came across so often during the walk.

The log was duly signed, and I was ready to begin the day's walking. First, however, I had to be driven back to the point where I had stopped walking on the previous day. At the exact spot, Harry dropped me off and drove back to Helmsdale to do a little shopping and wait for me to arrive.

It was by now about ten minutes after nine. It was still bright and sunny but the headwind was as strong as before. However, I felt very fit, and an hour and a half later I was back in Helmsdale. This first part of the day's programme was not a pleasure, it felt wrong somehow to be heading for the place I had left that morning! I made up my mind that it wouldn't happen again if it could be helped.

Once through Helmsdale, I felt better and even the wind had moderated a little. The countryside seemed more varied and interesting with a few trees and bushes providing a touch of green to brighten the grey landscape. I strode on, keeping up the rhythm of my steps and concentrating on the road beneath my feet. I was beginning to feel hungry and guessed it was nearly time to stop for lunch, when my progress was halted by my falling over something metal that lay in the gutter. I tripped and landed in a heap, but only my dignity was hurt. I discovered that I had stumbled over a rusted exhaust pipe that had separated itself from its parent vehicle.

The shock of the fall seemed to wake me up and trigger my senses, and it

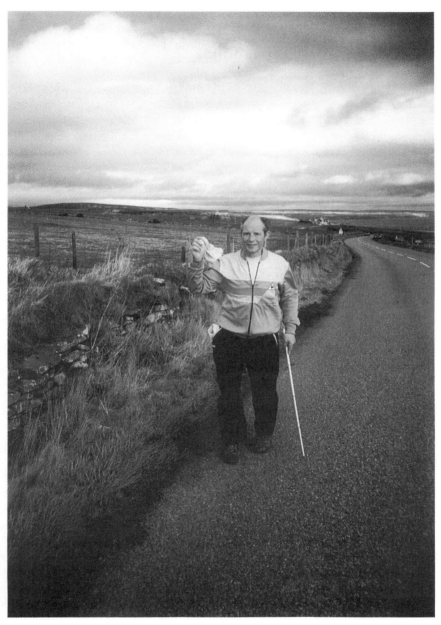

Blowing in the Wind (Scotland)

37

was then I realised that I had fallen into a kind of hypnotic trance from concentrating too closely and at one angle. After this I made a conscious effort to break my concentration and look up after every ten steps or so. Obviously I wasn't counting all the time, but from then on I was very conscious of the need to break my fixed stare at regular intervals as often as I could. I had to balance the danger of losing concentration and wandering into the road with the danger of hypnotising myself and slowing my reactions.

We stopped for lunch near Lothbeg, which was, like many other places we passed through merely half a dozen or so houses on either side of the road. Lunch consisted of the last of Mrs. Bremner's sandwiches which had remained remarkably fresh, a pork pie, coffee, and for dessert a generous square of "nutty slack". This crunchy biscuit type of cake has always been a favourite of mine, and Edna had made large quantities to keep us well supplied along the route.

I was near Brora when the sound of a horn attracted my attention to a large yellow vehicle which had stopped just in front of me. I didn't know what was happening until I heard a familiar voice and had my hand shaken warmly. I recognised Graham Scott, out friend and saviour from Inverness. He told me that he was taking a broken down car northwards on the back of a transporter. He asked when I expected to reach Inverness, and looked extremely doubtful when I said that I expected to be there by Thursday. He didn't think that I would cover 60 miles in two days. Nevertheless he told me that he was going to inform the people at the Moray Firth Radio Station about my walk, and tell them that I would be in Inverness on Thursday afternoon.

Shortly after Graham had left, the sky clouded over and down came the rain, driving into my face and in no time I was paddling in the stream flowing down the side of the road and my feet were soaked. The storm only lasted for about an hour, but it had been uncomfortable walking and although my feet were not cold or uncomfortable, they were very wet.

Past Dunrobin Castle through Golspie, and on to Cambusmore Lodge with Loch Fleet on my left, stretching for two miles until it joined the North Sea at a place called Littleferry. The countryside was less bleak than before. I was moving easily and keeping to my 4 mph so in spite of the wind and my wet feet, it was a good day. While I was walking I was calculating where I was; what time I could expect to be at other places along the route; how far I had come; how far I had to go and whether I was still on time. I was able to do this without it affecting my concentration.

My aim for the day was to get to Dornoch by six o clock . I had been making frequent stops for drinks, but they had been very brief and I was making good time. At five o clock Harry drove off to find somewhere for us to stay and soon returned to report his success. At six o clock I walked into Dornoch, feeling unreasonably pleased with myself, not at the distance walked, but because my calculations had worked out so precisely.

The place that Harry had found for us to stay for the night was a house belonging to Mrs. Matheson. She gave us a warm welcome, and showed us a large, comfortable room with two single beds. After making us a cup of tea to make us feel at home, she suggested a place where we could get an evening meal. I asked her about new bridge that was being built across Dornoch Firth. I had noticed that it was under construction when we had driven past on the way up, and I was holding out a hope that it might be usable. Mrs. Matheson didn't think that the work was complete yet, but she had read something in the local paper about a group of schoolchildren which had been taken across it, so she presumed that it must be nearly finished.

After a warm shower and a change of clothes, Harry and I decided to go and have a look at the new bridge, so we drove out about four miles to investigate. It seemed to be very near to completion, except for the section connecting the Northern approach road to the bridge, about 50 yards. This area was at this time simply mounds of earth, shuttering and concrete and there were ladders up the few feet to the bridge itself. I persuaded myself that I would be able to persuade the construction workers to let me across, since it would save about eight miles of walking. Without the bridge it is necessary to go round the Firth by way of Bonar Bridge.

We returned to Dornoch and made our telephone report home. There was still no news about a car and the caravanette had not yet returned. We followed Mrs. Matheson's advice and went to the Dornoch Hotel to eat. She had told us that if we sat in the bar instead of the dining room, we would get a good meal for about half the price. By now it was getting quite dark but following the directions we had been given, Harry found the way there. I recall climbing some stone steps and walking through a garden or park. I remember thinking that I would like to have seen more of Dornoch, since it impressed me as an attractive and interesting place.

The Hotel was warm and the atmosphere was friendly. We sat in the bar at a tablecloth covered table, had a drink, and ordered the roast of the day. This was duck served with all the trimmings and followed by a mouth watering sweet. It was a superb meal for which we were charged only £6.50p. We struck up a conversation with a fellow diner, who gave us a generous donation and added it to the money in the tin that someone had given to Harry during the day and I felt that it had been a satisfying and worthwhile day.

It was raining when we left the Hotel so the walk back was not so pleasant. After sorting out my wet boots and clothes I returned to my map. This time

I wanted to plan not only the next day's route, but also to work out when I could expect to reach Edinburgh, if I continued to cover an average of thirty miles each day. Harry was very dubious about my optimistic forecast, pointing out that we had to go through highland passes and may have to contend with worsening weather conditions. He also said that my initial enthusiasm might wear off. After voicing his provisos, Harry then admitted that he was beginning to realise that I would ignore adverse conditions, and overcome all but the most impossible problems and that we would probably reach Edinburgh exactly when I thought we would. This would be the ninth of April, according to my calculations, three days earlier than we had originally planned. My target for the following day was to get to the south of Alness. I needed to do this if I were to reach Inverness on Thursday as I had said to Graham Scott. I also wanted to give us a little time to do some fund raising in Inverness, since that, after all was the object of the walk. It was strange how the logistical problems of the walk, and the energy and drive needed to cover the distances seemed to take over, and it was easy to forget that the real aim of the whole thing was to collect money for Moorfields Hospital.

Day Four

I was up early, had breakfast at seven, and was on my way before eight. It was Wednesday 3rd of April. and as far as the weather was concerned, the best morning so far, bright sunny and cold. The wind was still from the south, but was not so strong. Harry soon caught up with me, having stayed behind to pay the bill, fill up the flask, get the log signed and collect some sandwiches that Mrs. Matheson had made for us. Once again the bill was lower than we would have expected!

I walked along the coast road towards the new bridge until I reached the approach road. This was only about half the distance we had travelled the previous evening when we had come through Evelix on a more inland route.

At the bridge I asked two men who were working there if it was alright to go across. They said that they would not stop me, but if the engineer saw me, he might. With that I climbed onto the bridge and started walking. It is quite a long bridge and there were vehicles on it so that I knew the southern end must be connected. I was half way over when a young fellow with an air of authority approached me. This was the engineer, who quite pleasantly, but firmly insisted that I went back the way I had come. On this occasion my soft soap didn't work at all. I tried asking him what he would have done if I had come from the south, and when he said he would have sent me back that way, I suggested that we swap places and he sent me back south. He smiled at this, but remained insistent. Back north I went, a wiser, but not particularly sadder man. As I passed the two workmen on the way off the bridge one of them sympathised with me, saying that he thought the engineer would be about. I was philosophical;

"Some you win, some you lose"

and this was just how I felt. There had always been the chance that the plan to cross the bridge would not come off. I had done a couple of miles extra, and had not saved the eight that I had hoped to save, but in the context of the whole undertaking, this was very little. Harry, who had been watching me intently all this time, was more upset than I was. He did agree with me however, that as the sun was out and we had a long way to go, we might as well get on with it.

The road along Dornoch Firth to Bonar Bridge had a good surface as far as I could tell, and I was able to keep up a good pace. After a while it clouded over but the rain held off until I had crossed the Bonar Bridge and

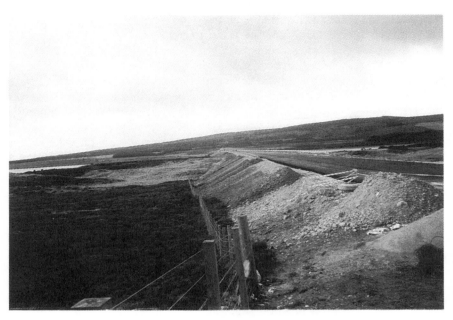

The Unfinished Bridge

turned east along the south side of the Dornoch Firth, through Kincardine, just before turning south onto the A836, the Struie Pass.

I had covered 16 miles in an untidy sort of way when I met up with Harry for a lunch break. There was another 14 miles to go to Alness. At this point it began to rain heavily, and we extended our lunch break to give it chance to ease off. There were a couple more heavy showers that day which did not last long, but they were a nuisance because of the time needed to put waterproofs on and off.

From the point at which I joined the A836 at Fearn Lodge to the Aultnamian Inn it was about 7 miles of uphill walking, some of it quite steep, but this was balanced by the next 7 miles to Alness, which was all downhill. When we reached Dalnavie, 3 miles north of Alness, Harry went on to find a B. & B. for the night. While studying the map I had realised that in fact Alness was bypassed by my route, but since we had previously decided that we would spend the night there, when I came to the road leading to the town, I followed it. I reached the town without meeting Harry, so I guessed that he had assumed that we would pass through the town on the A9 as we had on the journey north. However the A9 which follows the coast and avoids the ups and downs of the Struie Pass is fine for vehicles, but is in

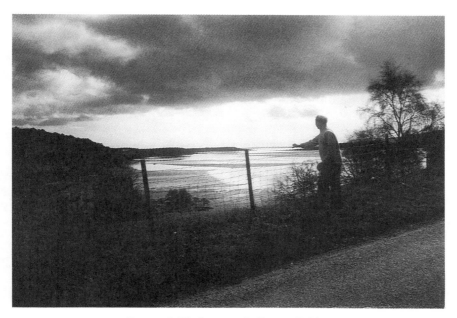

Dornoch Firth towards Bonar Bridge

fact 12 miles longer than the route I had chosen to walk. I now had to think about where I would be most likely to meet up with Harry. After walking around for a while I decided to wait on the most open part of the road. This was on the bridge over the River Averon, which would be a spot where I could be seen easily.

It wasn't long before Harry found me. He admitted that he hadn't studied the map, and assumed the route would be the same as before. He had found a room at a commercial inn which was situated to the south of Alness, and on the way to Inverness. I didn't want to travel to the inn by car, since it would mean backtracking the following day. I therefore walked the two miles to the inn so that I could get straight on with my journey in the morning.

The inn was an ordinary wayside pub. The room was clean and comfortable, and as we could get something to eat in the bar we were able to relax sooner, instead of having to go out to find something to eat. It had been nearly six o'clock when I had stopped walking, and I had travelled 32 miles. I was pleased that I had kept up with my schedule in spite of the detour in the morning, the delay because of the rain at lunch time, and the mix up over meeting Harry at Alness. I felt that it had been a satisfactory day's progress.

After a bath, I made my telephone call home. I used a pay phone which would not take incoming calls, and it seemed to be eating my coins. I tried to listen to what Edna was telling me while constantly feeding the telephone. I gathered that the caravanette had returned, a little the worse for wear with a few peripherals missing, like the spare wheel cover and the number plate! Also, Edna was optimistic that this time Rover really were going to provide a vehicle for some of the journey. I still had my doubts, since I had been disappointed before, but Harry was convinced that if anyone could persuade Rover to come up trumps, it would be Edna.

Harry read a notice in the inn which said that breakfast was available from six o'clock and anyone wanting a breakfast at that time should let them know the previous evening. I asked Harry to order a six o'clock breakfast for me, since that would give me the early start I needed if I were to get to Inverness in time to visit the radio station and then do some street collecting. Harry was a bit reluctant at first, but I explained that there was really no need for him to get up at that time, he could have his breakfast later and give me two or three hours start.

We had a very satisfying bar meal which was very good value. After a leisurely drink I went to our room to study the route for the following day. It wasn't long before it was clear in my mind, and then I went to bed early as I intended to be up by five thirty in the morning.

Day Five

I woke early and had no difficulty getting up in time for my breakfast at six. I was sitting in a little annexe by the kitchen taking in the appetising smells of my breakfast being prepared and drinking a cup of tea when two other guests came in , wished me good morning and sat down. Suddenly the proprietor, clearly angry, burst out of the kitchen and demanded to know what these two gentlemen were doing in the dining room at this time. Surprised, one of them explained that they would like breakfast. The proprietor informed them that they should have ordered it the previous evening, so they apologised and explained that it had been late when they booked in, they had gone straight to bed and they hadn't seen the notice. The proprietor was purple with rage, he demanded that they clear off out of his hotel, he didn't want them or their money. he wanted them off the premises immediately, they need not pay for their room. He accused them of being English and taking jobs from Scots people, and was extremely offensive.

The two men stood up, thanked him and walked out, leaving him absolutely fuming. Long after they had gone he was still muttering about the English, and that Scotland should be for the Scots not foreigners. I did point out to him that I was English, but thought it better not to argue with him and did not elaborate about the Scots who I had worked with and who were my friends in England and who had experienced no such prejudice. The food, I suppose, was alright but it was impossible for me to enjoy it in such an atmosphere. I ate my breakfast and got away as soon as I could, but the unpleasantness of this incident stayed with me for some time. Whatever it was that had got into this man, there can be no excuse for such behaviour, and it came as such a contrast to all the other friendly, helpful and pleasant people we had met. Mrs. Matheson for instance, who as well as all her kindness, had put a generous donation in our tin as we came away. That man is the only person I came across on the whole journey that I wouldn't want to meet again, even the engineer who had refused to let me cross the bridge had done so politely, and he was only doing his job, no doubt if I had had an accident on the unfinished bridge he would have had to take the responsibility for allowing me to be there. I could see now that I had been thoughtless in trying to persuade him to change his mind.

Anyway, its an ill wind that does no good at all, and it did get me out quickly. I was walking before half past six. There was still a light southerly wind and a damp mist but nothing that would slow me down. It was April 4th and I aimed to reach Daviot, just south of Inverness. This meant a day's walk of 26 miles which was far enough if I was to do all the other things that were planned for the day. It was after 9 o'clock when Harry caught up with me and I had walked 10 miles and was ready for a drink. Walking is very thirsty work. I had found that between breakfast and lunch I didn't eat but needed to drink regularly, not much at a time, but often. After lunch I still needed to take frequent small drinks, usually fruit juice, but I also tended to eat a little, a biscuit or a piece of chocolate.

While I was having a drink I told Harry about the behaviour of the hotel proprietor at breakfast. Harry hadn't had any trouble after I left, the man had signed the log, but had said that he was too busy to fill our flask. Harry had returned to Alness to get the flask filled and had also bought some sandwiches and a postcard. We were trying to send a postcard home each day as a record of the journey.

We had crossed the Cromarty Firth and were now on the Black Isle. This is a pleasant rolling agricultural area with plenty of trees and livestock, and I felt quite at home walking in such an environment. The A9 was busy but the going was easy and I had crossed the Moray Firth and walked up the long hill on the road south that bypasses Inverness before I stopped for lunch. When we had had something to eat, as we were within about 4 miles of the target destination, Harry went off to find somewhere for us to stay that night. I reached Daviot by 2 o'clock and found Harry waiting for me at the top of a steep hill that led into the village. He had booked us into a small boarding house which was an attractive building in a lovely setting and which provided an evening meal which was another bonus for us. However we did not stay there long enough to appreciate it at this stage, for after a shower and a change of clothes we were on our way back to Inverness to try and find the Moray Firth Radio station. We were very fortunate that the first person we asked knew where it was and gave us clear directions that Harry was able to follow. It is amazing how difficult it usually is to find someone to give directions who is not either a complete stranger to the area or quite unable to tell their left from their right. We found the radio station at about half past three and after introducing ourselves, we were taken through a large desk lined office to a small room where a man was sitting in front of a console. He was pressing buttons and turning knobs while talking at an amazing speed that I have only heard beaten by cattle auctioneers. The fast-talking, apparently ambidextrous DJ seemed to disappear however when he put on a record, took off his headphones and gave us a relaxed smile. He knew who we were and what we were doing since Graham Scott had told him about us and we were expected. In a surprisingly quietly spoken voice, he guided me through an interview in a situation which would normally have found me nervous and tongue-tied. In answer to his skilful questions I was able to explain the object of the walk, and also that I would be in Inverness with my collecting tin later that afternoon.

It was cold and damp standing in Inverness, but the generosity and friendliness of the people made what would normally have been a chore into a pleasant experience. After an hour and a half of collecting I was ready to leave the almost empty town centre and to return to the boarding house for my meal. It was now about six thirty p.m. A man had just put some money in my tin and walked away. After about half a dozen steps he turned, came back and said;

"You look cold, have a dram on me" and put £1.00 in my pocket,
As he did this, another man, making a donation , also gave me £1.00,
saying;
"Have one on me as well"

My face must have shown the surprise and gratitude that I was too cold to express, for they walked off together, laughing.

We returned to the Guest house in a good mood. Harry had not done any of the collecting, but had helped with changing the tins when they got too heavy (£20 00 in coins can weigh. heavily) and had managed to get me a warm cup of tea which had been a great help.

There was a telephone box in the village so making our call home was no problem. The news was good; Rover were providing us with a car for two weeks from the 10th April. My replanned schedule would get me to Edinburgh on the ninth, and although I did not really want a wait of two days, it would give me a chance to do some collecting. Edna said she would organise the changeover of drivers and arrange for the person who was coming to Edinburgh to take Harry home to meet us there. The arrangements were beginning to fall into place.

The meal we had that evening was not large, but it was tasty, and well prepared and served. Afterwards we sat in the Lounge with the other guests, a couple from Glasgow and a family from Minnesota, U.S.A. and had a pleasant evening. At about ten o'clock I retired to study my map and decide where the next day's walk should end. 30 miles would get me to Kincraig, so that was to be my target. It had been a thoroughly satisfying day, easy walking, a good collection, good food and lodgings and pleasant company.

Day Six

Friday, 5th April. Breakfast at 7.30 was again not large, but well-cooked and enjoyable. The proprietors were talkative but nevertheless businesslike. They presented the bill before we sat down, and had made us sandwiches and filled our flask as we had asked. I was on the road by 8 o'clock and soon I was passing the place where we had broken down last Saturday. As I passed the small, peaceful cafe with its adjoining forecourt and petrol pumps, I thought of the pushing, shoving and frustration of that exhausting few hours Less than six days ago , so much seemed to have happened since then!

Harry had some shopping to do, and also decided to do a little sight-seeing since we were very close to the site of the battlefield of Culloden Muir or Moor south east of Inverness. This suited me, as I liked two or three hours of uninterrupted early morning walking. The morning began fine. Just before lunch, a squall hit me; the wind rose, the sky turned black and hail fell like chips of glass on my face. It only lasted about half an hour but it was enough to turn the hills white. The higher peaks were well covered with snow and I could understand why this was a popular winter sports area.

I stopped for lunch just north of Carbridge. I had travelled 17 miles, and with only 13 miles to go to Kincraig, I thought we would have time to do an hour's collecting in Aviemore. It would mean a short diversion, but we were interested to see what Aviemore was like. When we arrived we were not very impressed. There was one main road with a few shops, mainly gift shops and sports shops as one would expect in a holiday centre, but there didn't seem to be any life in the place. The few people about seemed fed up and bored, probably since by this time it was quite windy and there was a miserable drizzle. I did try to do a little collecting, and people gave generously, but there were so few of them that I gave up after about three quarters of an hour and decided to press on and cover the six miles left to go before Kincraig.

Shortly after I restarted my walk, Harry drove off to Kincraig in order to organise accommodation. We had left the A9 to go into Aviemore, and we were now on the B9152. This runs parallel to the A9 and does not bypass Kincraig. This had the advantages of being a quieter road, and also that I could continue along it to Kincraig without having to look for turn-offs.

Harry was waiting when I reached Kincraig. He had found a comfortable place for us to stay and had been told where we could get an evening meal. It was nearly six o'clock when I finally completed my target for the day and

I felt that it had been a long day. The walking had not been hard, and I had covered the 30 miles, but I decided that it was not a good idea to break a walk in order to collect.

A relaxing bath and a change of clothes helped me to feel more positive. My telephone call to Edna brought news that Rover had confirmed the arrangement to loan us a car for two weeks from the 11th April. The car would be delivered to my next driver's house on the tenth. I was confident of reaching Edinburgh on the afternoon of the 9th April since I had managed to keep up with my self-imposed schedule up to this point. In telling Edna this, however, I was committing myself to maintaining my fairly punishing schedule since she would now go ahead and make the arrangements with the people who had offered us accommodation in Edinburgh and with the driver who was coming to take Harry back home. All I had to do was to make sure that we could cover the next 125 miles in under 4 days !! I already had a rough mental picture of the route I would take, and how it would break down, but I would have to work it out in detail later that evening. First and most important, though was our need for food. We had been told of a good restaurant a mile or so along the road and we drove through the evening drizzle to find an attractive wooden building on the edge of an attractive lake, Lake Insh. The daylight was beginning to go, but I was still able to appreciate that I was in a place of remarkable, peaceful beauty. The restaurant was called 'The Boathouse' and I think it must have been built on a promontory. Harry and I were shown to a table overlooking the water, and as the waitress led the way, walked into a chair and knocked it over. Harry apologised on my behalf, explaining that I could not see. The waitress was very understanding, and admitted that she too had a problem with her eyesight.

The Restaurant was quite full. There were several groups of winter sports enthusiasts and there was a cheerful atmosphere in the place. The food both looked and tasted first class and we really indulged ourselves, ordering a three course meal and coffee. We spent a little more than we had budgeted for, but we felt entitled to allow ourselves a little luxury. So far things were going so well. I was covering the miles without any real discomfort or difficulty despite the bad weather. In our ignorance and in self-congratulatory mood, we wrongly assumed that the weather could only improve from this point; it certainly didn't occur to us that it could get any worse.

After we had eaten, the waitresses spoke to us about the walk and asked us to explain more about the Fight for Sight Campaign. One of the girl's told us that she was a student at Edinburgh University who was working at the restaurant during the Spring Recess. She revealed that she too had a problem with her eyes for which she was hoping to get some treatment. As far as I could see her eyes looked perfect with all the sparkle and attractiveness of youth, so her disability was not at all obvious and I did not ask for details. However I hope she has had her treatment, and that it has been successful.

We paid our bill and promised to send them a postcard from Land's End. As we left, they put a generous donation in our collecting tin, this was the more appreciated since it was from young people who were working through their holidays in order to make ends meet.

Then it was back to the B & B, where I did my nightly map study and Harry arranged with Mrs. Neck, the Landlady, for a filled flask and sandwiches for the following day.

Day Seven

Saturday morning was dry and bright and I was feeling very bright as I set off just after eight o'clock. A good night's sleep and a big breakfast had put me in the mood to go far and fast. It was not long, however, before driving rain and a strong headwind changed my feeling of optimistic enthusiasm to one of dogged determination to survive the day and achieve my target. By the time I reached Kingussie two hours later I was more than pleased to meet up with Harry and to stop for a warm drink.

Soon after, the rain turned to sleet which was being driven into my face by the strong wind. In order to lessen the discomfort, it was necessary for me to put my head down, and thus reduce the area of my vision. As a result, I found that I was stepping on, or stumbling over a large number of things that lay on the roadside where I walked. There were small animals and birds, killed by the traffic and what seemed like vast amounts of debris that must have flown off passing vehicles. There were bits of exhausts, wing mirrors, and pieces of rubber from tyres, some of which were a yard or so long. It is quite frightening to think of what could have happened if a lorry had passed me with a piece of its tyre flailing about, or hurling a detached mirror in my direction! At the time, however, I was not bothered by such thoughts for I was much too busy concentrating on simply keeping going.

It was commonplace to trip over the body of a rabbit which had foolishly ventured onto the highway, and later that day there were white hares as well. I was surprised by the large numbers of game birds and birds of prey which had shared a similar fate. I was told that the birds of prey gorge themselves, and then become too heavy and slow to dodge the traffic.

I left Kingussie and made my way along the A9 bypassing Newtonmore; through Etteridge towards Dalwhinnie. Glen Truim and the River Truim were on my right hand side, but I didn't see either. At least here the walking was reasonably level and despite the oncoming sleet which was now turning to snow, I was making satisfactory progress.

I stopped for a lunch break about a mile to the north of Dalwhinnie. By this time Harry was concerned about the increasingly bad weather, as he thought it impossible for me to be seen by passing motorists. I was determined to get through the Drumochter Pass before I gave in. This involved a climb to 2,500 feet and I didn't want that at the start of a day. I was also very unwilling to get so far behind my schedule.

I started off again. By now the temperature had dropped considerably and I soon had to stop in order to put on my gloves and woollen hat under

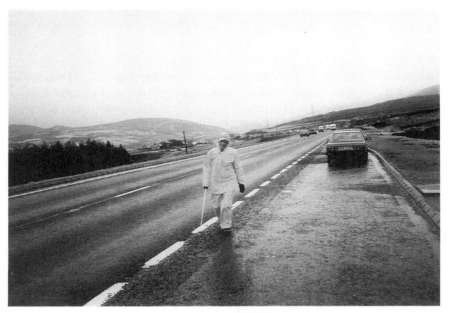

Foul Weather Approaching Drummochter

my waterproofs. These kept most of my body quite warm and dry. Even my feet felt warm, although my boots were full of water and I could feel it oozing out over the tops with every step. My fingers and face were the exception and were suffering from the cold. Every vehicle that passed sent a spray of dirty white slush in my direction.

It is a long climb from Dalwhinnie through the Drumochter Pass and as I cleared the snow from my eyes and saw it caking on my front it seemed like very slow going. However, a later reckoning showed that I had kept up a good speed. It should have been a demoralising and uncomfortable time, but in fact I didn't feel tired and was rather enjoying the struggle against the adverse conditions. I felt as if I were an Arctic explorer battling against the elements and when I said this to Harry, he replied that in my bright yellow waterproofs I looked more like a lump of iced custard floating around in the gutter. He was still worried about my being seen as he felt sure that drivers already contending with snow on their windscreens would have their visibility greatly reduced. He would not therefore go on ahead to find somewhere to stay but preferred to stay as close as possible. I understood his concern and as we had by this time come through the Drumochter Pass I agreed that I would stop when I reached Dalnacardoch Lodge which is at the end of the dual carriageway through the Glen Garry that I had now reached and about 5 miles north of Calvin.

I had passed signs which would have told me that I was reaching particular high points along the way, but even if the conditions had been more favourable, I would not have stopped to try and make out the details. At a point about three miles short of Dalnacardoch Lodge, I stopped at a convenient lay-by and to Harry's relief agreed that in such conditions, the 29 miles that I had covered was far enough.

We drove into Calvin and booked in at the Struan Inn for B & B. However, considering the day we had had, we were thankful that they also provided an evening meal which meant we did not have to venture out again. First, though I needed a bath, a change of clothes, a cup of tea, and then a telephone to report our progress.

I had stopped walking at about half past five , so although it had taken me longer than i had anticipated to cover the distance, I had managed to keep up a speed of around three and a half mph. Nevertheless I had not reached my target for the day, and still had over 90 miles to go before I reached Edinburgh.

Edna needed a reasonably accurate estimate of the time I would expect to reach Edinburgh, as there were still things she needed to arrange. I did not want to tell her how far I still had to go since I was still determined to make it to Edinburgh within three days. I said that I would work out the timing, and tell her the following evening what my E.T.A at Queensferry would be. Queensferry is over the bridge and on the Edinburgh side of the Firth of Forth. Edna accepted this, and demonstrated a faith in my planning that was as strong as my faith in hers. She remarked that the weather reports on the television had shown that the weather in Scotland was not very good. I agreed that it wasn't, without going into more detail, and when I told Harry this at dinner, he nearly choked. Whatever he thought of my skill as a walker, he had boundless admiration for my skill as master of the understatement.

The meal was a good one, well prepared and generous in portion. After a drink in the pleasant and congenial atmosphere of the pub. Lounge, it was easy to relax and forget the rigours of the day, well almost! After this we retired, Harry with his book, and me with my maps. We had now been travelling south for six and a half days and had covered 200 miles with no aches and pains, no blisters and only one real problem- that of getting my boots and socks dry. The socks I was able to put on a radiator with my hat and gloves, and they would be dry by the morning. The boots were more of a problem. I had changed boots twice during the day, which I now realised was a serious mistake, because I now had three pairs of wet boots, which even when stuffed with paper and put as near to the radiators as I dare without risk to the leather would still be damp the next morning. This meant that I would have wet feet the next day even if the weather were dry. Another lesson learned!

I decided that the next day I should reach Dunkeld if I was to keep up the schedule I had set for myself. This meant I had to walk an ambitious 34 miles which I knew I could do if I could get an early start. This would be a problem because the earliest breakfast was not served until half past eight. Harry, good old Harry, agreed to get up early and drive me back to the lay-by where I had stopped walking. This meant that I could complete the first part of that day's walk and arrive back at the hotel in time for breakfast. It might seem a crazy way to carry on, but I was determined that every step of the way should be covered with no short-cuts... and besides, I wasn't going to miss out on an excellent breakfast!

We took care to forewarn our hosts of the plan, so that if they heard us creeping out in the early morning, they would not think we were trying to avoid paying the bill.

Day Eight

Six o'clock found me up and about, refreshed after a good night's sleep. Harry was not so lively but after a cup of tea he rallied round and we were soon on our way to the lay-by where yesterday's walk had ended. The weather was still rather grim but when I set out in the cold, sleety rain I was relieved to discover that the wind had veered and was now coming from the west. This was a distinct improvement because I could now direct my eyes forward and this widened the field of my vision.

At six-thirty I began to walk, and at eight o'clock I was back at the Struan Inn in time to dry off before breakfast. Although my feet were damp from wearing wet boots, at least no more water had got in them. Perhaps the conditions were not so wet, and I had noticed that there was much less traffic on the road, which eased things considerably. This was probably due both to my early start and to the fact that today was Sunday.

Breakfast over, and I was on my way again. Harry stayed behind to put our things back in the car, pay the bill, and get the log signed and dated. I passed through Pitagowan, Blair Atholl and the Pass of Killycrankie. The rain had eased to little more than a drizzle and with the wind not nearly so unfriendly as it had been on the day before, I was making good progress. It was also considerably warmer and I was sweating under my waterproofs, which acted as wind cheaters. This had not happened yesterday, when the colder weather had kept my body temperature about right. It proves that it is indeed an ill wind the does no good at all!

Harry caught up with me just as I was passing through Blair Atholl. He was much happier for me today with the better visibility, the lighter traffic and the more even terrain. It was much easier for him to keep an eye on me. I continued along the winding road that follows the course of the river Garry and which crosses and recrosses the river on the Pass of Killycrankie and then bypasses Pitlochrie, and then stopped for lunch only twelve miles north of the day's target, Dunkeld.

During lunch, the rain stopped and I was able to discard my waterproofs when I set off again on the last few miles of that day's schedule. The rest of the journey was pleasantly uneventful. At four o'clock, and about four miles from Dunkeld, Harry went on ahead to do his usual chore of finding us somewhere to stay for the night. We arranged to meet at the junction of the A9 and the road off that goes east for half a mile to the town. Harry met me as arranged, and as he had left the car in town, we walked together into Dunkeld which is a small cathedral town with old, grey stone buildings with a peaceful atmosphere which appealed to me. We were to stay in an old house in the Cathedral Close with a Mrs. Sheret, who made us feel very welcome, ushering us into the sitting room where she had a pot of tea and a plate of freshly baked cakes laid out for us. To our surprise she said that she had been expecting us, for a friend of hers who had stayed with her the previous evening had seen me on the Drumochter Pass and had told her that at the speed I was travelling I would be in Dunkeld by Sunday evening. The friend had also described to her the dreadful weather, saying that it was the worst they had seen that winter, all this making me feel that perhaps I wasn't doing too badly so far. Mrs Sheret had to go out that evening, but she told us where we could eat and made sure that we had a key and that we were comfortable and had everything we needed to make ourselves feel at home. We were in no hurry to eat, so after a bath and a change of clothes I decided to do a little bit of planning so that I could give Edna some times for my arrival at Queensferry.

According to my reckoning we were about fifty miles from Queensferry and it was about another twelve miles from there to the place where we had been invited to stay in Edinburgh. I therefore decided to aim for Kinross which was thirty one miles away, and this would leave me about the same distance to cover on the following day. I calculated that I should reach Queensferry at two o'clock on Tuesday. This calculation left no margin for error or setbacks, but I was confident that it would work out.

I explained the details to Edna when I telephoned and she was able to inform me that the organisers of The Fight for Sight Campaign had arranged for representatives of the media to meet me, and also, which was much better news from my point of view, that she had had an offer from the brother of one of our neighbours, a schoolteacher in Edinburgh, to meet me at Queensferry and walk with me to the flat in which we were to stay. This was very good news, because I had not been looking forward to finding my way through Edinburgh. Now Edna could go ahead and tell the person who was coming to take Harry home from Edinburgh exactly when we would be there. Wilf Barnett, who was to be my next guardian would meet me at the flat on Thursday, providing Rover delivered the car to him on Wednesday, as promised.

Everything seemed to be working out. I wasn't enthusiastic about being interviewed by the media, but our experience in Inverness had shown how the publicity had helped when it came to collecting money, and as I intended to spend my 'waiting' day collecting in Edinburgh, I resolved to do the best I could.

We were fortunate to have a little time to look around Dunkeld, a pleasant stroll round a quiet, old town. There was little traffic and the atmosphere reminded me of Sundays as I remembered them of fifty or more years ago. We found the restaurant that Mrs. Sheret had spoken of and found the food to be good, and as usual in Scotland, very substantial. During the meal we discussed the best way to approach the next two days. Harry suggested that if I wanted an early start, he could pick me up before breakfast and drive me back to Mrs. Sheret's to eat, and then return me to the point I had reached. This seemed a splendid idea to me for two reasons. Firstly I liked walking early when the roads are quieter, and secondly, I enjoyed my food more after I had had some exercise. With this in mind we returned to our lodgings. Again I made a careful study of the next day's route before turning in for an early night.

Day Nine

Six o'clock on Monday, 8th April. I set off in heavy rain heading towards Perth. While there was not much traffic about, there was enough to get me well sprayed and my feet soaked. It is not the rain coming down that wets my feet but the spray that goes over the top of my boots and the puddles I walk through without knowing that they are there. On through Birnam, along the road following the course of the River Isla until after three miles the river turns east. I continued south through the Muir of Thorn and Bankfoot and I was approaching Luncarty when Harry caught up with me. He had been growing very anxious, thinking that I could not possibly have walked so far, and he had been on the point of turning back in case he had passed me. It was a quarter past eight and I had walked nine miles.

We were soon back in Dunkeld enjoying the enormous breakfast that Mrs. Sheret had set out for us. My early morning walking had done wonders for my appetite. Mrs. Sheret told us about her daughter, now living in Canada, who was born blind due to an excess of oxygen. I was able to tell her that Professor Ashton, the Chairman of the Fight for Sight Campaign is the person who discovered the role of excess oxygen as the cause of blindness in premature babies. His study, carried out at Moorfields Hospital had prevented a situation which had been responsible for approximately 7,000 babies each year being born blind.

The rain had eased considerably in the hour or so since I had returned to Dunkeld, so, despite my resolution to the contrary I indulged in the luxury of putting on dry boots and socks, and after getting the log signed and collecting a flask of hot coffee and a packed lunch we were on our way once again. It was a quarter to ten when we reached the place where Harry had caught up with me. The rain had stopped and there was even a little brave hint of sunshine for which I was grateful. The real pleasure at this point was in being able to walk without waterproofs.

Soon Lucarty was behind me and I crossed the River Almond near Scone Palace and then to Perth, going east of the town centre before weaving under and over motorways and eventually reaching the A912 at Craigend continuing for another mile south to Kintille, where we stopped for lunch. As things were going so well and I believed that I was only about twelve miles from Kinross, I suggested that we travel on secondary roads for the rest of that day. I had studied this alternative route, and decided that although it wasn't any further, it would probably take longer. It would be good to have a break from the heavy traffic. Harry was all for it as if anyone needed to get away from the constant stream of traffic for a while, then he did! So off we went, and what a pleasure it was to be able to look about me at the fields and hedges of this rolling countryside so green and peaceful that it reminded me of my daily walks at home. We crossed under, and then over, the M90 that was never very far away, but in atmosphere we were so remote from it that it could have been a different world. As we crossed over the motorway, I stopped to look at the twin conveyor belts of traffic going north and south; an utter contrast to the nine cars and two tractors that had passed me during the last two hours. Through the hamlets of Glenfarg and Duncrievie I went before turning on to the B996 and walking the last three miles into Kinross where Harry was waiting to direct me to the house where we were to stay that night. He had gone on when we reached the B996 to find a suitable place.

It was only half past four and I had covered thirty miles. It had been the easiest day so far. Mrs Barnes, at whose house we were staying, made us very welcome and told us that we would be able to get a good meal at the pub. opposite, but that would be later. I had time for a leisurely bath before changing into fresh clothes and going for a stroll around Kinross and finding a telephone so that I could pass on the news of a successful and enjoyable day's progress. The arrangements for our arrival in Edinburgh had been made. There was apparently to be quite a reception for us at Queensferry. My part in it was to be a simple one, I just had to be there at two o'clock. Charles Morrish, my guide to my temporary home in Edinburgh, Jean Eckington, who was to take Harry home were to be there at two; the Fight for sight Charity organisers had told Edna that they had arranged for the local media to be there also, but that it had to be at two o'clock, and not before or after! I still had nearly twenty miles to go, and I wondered if they realised how difficult it might become to keep such an appointment when almost anything could happen to delay us, the most likely problem would be bad weather. however, I had always expressed confidence that I could carry out my plan and perhaps it was my own fault that so much was expected of me. Harry had no doubt that I would be there spot on time.

The food at the pub was very good, and it proved my theory that local recommendation is a surer guide then any of the more famous published ones. We were also able to enjoy a drink and a chat with the people in the bar. They were interested in what we were doing and wanted to know all the details. It seems that almost everyone we talked to either had eye problems themselves, or knew someone who did, and as well as good wishes and encouragement, we were given a generous donation for the collecting tin.

After a brief look at my map, I went to bed at about ten o'clock. This morning's pre-breakfast start had been so successful that I wanted to use it as a pattern for the rest of the trip, and aimed to set off as early as possible.

Day Ten

Shortly after six the next morning, Tuesday 9th saw me striding out along the B996 out of Kinross towards Edinburgh. It was a fine, cool morning but with a strong south westerly wind which was doing its best to blow me back to John O'Groats. I was thankful that I did not need waterproofs, which billow out and making walking into the wind extremely hard going, nevertheless such a strong headwind was bound to take the edge off my speed. I had only walked about seven miles when Harry came for me at eight o'clock but it was enough for me to remain confident that I would get to Queensferry at the appointed hour. Mrs. Barnes proved to be the equal of our other Scottish landladies in the high quality and generous quantity of the breakfast she provided.

Thus well fed and full of confidence, I set off on the final leg of this first, and in many ways, the most difficult phase of the journey. If to me this day's progress signified the end of a stage of the whole enterprise, then to Harry it would mean the last of his eleven day ordeal, a period of unrelenting worry and responsibility which he had met with strength. His selflessness and conscientiousness during this time was amazing.

The road was fairly quiet , mainly, I suppose, because most of the traffic was using the M90 which ran parallel to the road we were on. I made steady progress along the B917 to Crossgates and then the B981 led us to the Forth Road Bridge, between Rosythe and Inverkeithing. The most memorable thing about this part of the walk, for me was the terrible state of the pavements in the villages that I walked through. How an elderly person, or anyone infirm could manage them is beyond me, and I'm sure that it would be impossible to push a pram or pushchair over such uneven surfaces. This, of course, may explain the dearth of pedestrians. After stumbling several times and falling once, I kept to the road.

I stopped about a mile north of the approach to the Forth Bridge. It was only just after twelve, but we decided to have our lunch. There were four miles to go to Queensferry, and I calculated that if I set off again at ten minutes before one o'clock, I should be able to time my arrival for two o'clock. Harry would drive across and meet me at the southern side of the bridge.

At twelve fifty prompt, we set off to make our separate crossings of the Firth of Forth. If I had judged the wind to be strong on the approach, then on the bridge itself it was mighty. I realised that it was slowing me down considerably, and began to wonder if I had left myself enough time.

Resurfacing work was taking place on the bridge and the traffic was merely crawling along. I kept passing and repassing the same vehicles, and one driver called to ask if I wanted a lift.

"No thanks" I said, "I'm in a hurry"
he roared with laughter as I walked on.

At two minutes to two I walked up the steps on to the car park at the Queensferry end of the bridge, to a tumultuous reception! Well, Harry, who was the only person there, clapped and cheered and asked me to say a few words into the microphone, masquerading as a plastic cup. Just as I was thanking the public, in the form of Harry, for its welcome and support, a minibus and car pulled up and twelve teenage girls and two adults emerged. For a brief moment, I wondered exactly what had been planned for me - and then I was introduced to Charles Morrish, a teacher at Firhill Secondary School, a colleague of his, and twelve of the students. They told me that their school was adjacent to a school for the blind, and Charles Morrish's colleague was in charge of the project which involved these girls in working with and assisting the blind students.

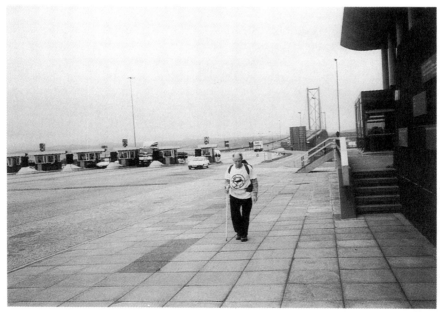

Arriving at Queensferry

While all this was happening, I noticed that the car driver was Jean Eckington. She had stopped outside the school to ask the way, and by coincidence had asked Charles, hence they had arrived together. She then went with Harry to Edinburgh Airport where they were to return the hire car. However, they were both coming back to stay at the flat before going home the next day.

After Jean and Harry had set off, one of the girls asked me what I had been doing when they arrived at the car park. I was puzzled at first, until I remembered that I had been waving my arms about and talking into a cup held in front of my face by Harry. I gave her this explanation, but I'm not sure that she was convinced by it!

It was quarter past two when we set off to walk the rest of the way in to Edinburgh. The girls walked with me, asking me questions which I did my best to answer. They were delightful company and I thought perhaps they had been specially selected, but I was assured that this was not so. There had been no sign of anyone from the press and I must confess that I was relieved rather than disappointed.

After an hour and a half, the girls boarded their minibus, which had been accompanying us and Charles, who was now my companion and I were able to set up a smarter pace. It was about half past five when we arrived at the flat which is situated Southeast of the town centre. Harry and Jean had arrived before us and had already introduced themselves to our hosts, Steffi and Colin. Before Charles left he asked me if I would be prepared to talk to the students at the school on Thursday morning before I set off on the next part of my walk. I agreed, in spite of the fact that I found the thought almost more daunting than the whole undertaking altogether! Charles was to telephone me to confirm the arrangement the next day.

I now had a little time to talk to my hosts. I had not met Colin before, but I knew Steffi, who is the daughter of a friend and neighbour. They could not have been more kind and helpful. The flat is not a very large one, but they managed to, accommodate three single guests and all the luggage from the hire car. They also supplied us with a very good dinner and breakfast.

Jean had brought a set of fresh clothes for me and would take the others back home. She would also take all the money we had collected so far and things that experience had shown we didn't need. Colin left after dinner to catch a train to Swansea where he had a meeting. I think he may have been to pleased to escape from the chaos we had brought to his home.

There was no route to study that evening, but there was a lot of sorting out to do because Jean and Harry wanted to set off as early as they could the next morning. I had telephoned Edna and told her about the day's events. She was annoyed that no-one from the media had turned up at Queensferry, as they had been most insistent on knowing the exact time that I would arrive there. This did not really matter to me, I was much more interested to hear that the Rover Company had confirmed that they would be delivering a car to Wilf Barnett at his home on Wednesday, and that he would get to me in Edinburgh some time during Thursday afternoon. That timetable meant that I now had a day and a half to use before I could set out on the next leg of the walk. I had already decided to spend the next day collecting in the city, and part of Thursday would be taken up by my visit to the school. I also hoped to find some time to walk to the outskirts of Edinburgh, to give myself as good a start as possible. Ideally I would want to get out of the built up area for when Wilf, my new driver arrived, he would find it easier to keep an eye on me out of the town, besides which, my progress is slower and I would be happier when that part of the walk was behind me.

Edna was pleased that we had managed to co-ordinate things so well at this stage, and that our plans and organisation were working out. She even asked me to estimate the point that I would have reached by Friday, 19th May, in ten days time, when the next change of driver was due. I told her that I wanted to be as near to Shrewsbury as possible, but that it was really far too early to commit myself.

In spite of the hectic day we had had, we nevertheless sat talking until quite late. It was a pleasant feeling to relax in good company. Steffi, who is a hydro-electrical engineer, told us that she would be away from home for the next three days, working in the north of Scotland and that I was nevertheless welcome to stay. She then thoughtfully showed me where things were in the kitchen. This was very useful, and I thanked her, but it didn't do much to ease my apprehension. I was to be on my own in a strange flat in a strange city and even in my home if something is moved a few inches from its familiar position, I can't find it. I resolved to keep calm and do everything slowly. The thought that I might cause some damage worried me, but I didn't say anything and eventually we retired to the various places were we were to sleep.

Day Eleven

It was a short night, we were all up and about early the next morning. Steffi left shortly after eight and I helped Jean and Harry to pack the car. This involved us all making three journeys out to where the car was parked from the third floor flat, and took some time. By nine o'clock they were on their way home, leaving me to return to the empty flat feeling a little low-spirited. Another cup of tea soon put me right and I prepared to go out with my collecting tins. Just before I left, there was a telephone call from Charles Morrish who said he would pick me up at half past eight the following morning to take me to school to talk to the students.

I made my way to the local shopping centre, remembering the directions which Colin had carefully given me. I took care to memorise the route so that I would be able to find my way back as well. Standing outside in the wind to collect money was uncomfortable, but people were generous and I stayed there for about three hours until it started to rain and I decided to take a break and find somewhere to have some lunch. During this time I was twice asked to show my permit to collect. In my experience this is unusual, and I was pleased to be able to show my credentials, since if this happened more it would cut down the numbers of bogus collectors who support only one cause, themselves!

I found my way to a nearby restaurant after taking off my Campaign T-shirt and putting it with the collecting tins into my rucksack. When I entered the restaurant, I stood for a little while just inside the door, trying to get my sight accustomed to the gloom and to get my bearings. I must have looked a bit lost, for I heard a quiet female voice asking if she could help. I told her that I wanted a meal, and she led me to a table and went off to find a waitress, who, when she came, told me what was on the menu without any fuss and made sure that I had everything I needed, even to telling me that the salt was on the right and the pepper on the left. After I had eaten and paid, the same waitress led me to the door, and wished me a good day and thanked me for my custom. I have no idea what either of these two ladies look like but I can still remember their voices and the thoughtful and discreet ways in which they helped me.

I walked back to the flat through the drizzle and rain and I was tempted to give up for the day, but it was too early for that. I changed over the collecting tins for empty ones and set off again, this time to the city centre, to Princes Street in the shadow of the Castle. The last time I had been there had been more than thirty years before on a family camping holiday. Although my eyesight was not a problem then, I can remember little about that fortnight we spent in Scotland, except that it rained for most of the time.

My collecting effort that afternoon was not very successful. There were not many people about, and those that were seemed in a hurry to get indoors. Willpower rather than enthusiasm kept me there for about three hours, before I retraced my carefully noted and remembered way back to the flat. Judging by the weight of the tins, there was more in them than I had thought but as it was my policy to open the tins only when someone was there to witness the amount as it was counted and recorded along with the number on the tin, it was sometime before I knew that I had collected over £100 on that day. At the time I felt quite low and depressed, feeling that this time was an unwanted delay from the real task in hand, which was to get on with the walk.

Back at the flat there was a number of things I had to do. I wanted to have all the things that would go with us packed so that I knew where they were, and so that they were convenient to get at. Then there was the route to study. I spent a long time poring over the road map of Edinburgh, lent to me by Charles. I had to be sure of finding my way to the outskirts, and since I would not have a driver to bring me back, I had to be equally sure of finding my way back. I also had my regular telephone report to make.

I had time to take stock of my surroundings, and from the elevated position of the flat, there were good views of the city, and the Castle was clearly visible. To me Edinburgh is a place of interest and character, where the people had been kind and generous but nevertheless the sooner I was on my way, the happier I would be.

The packing took longer than I had anticipated. I would get so far, and then find something else that ought to be packed underneath what had already been done. I had managed to do most of the work, and stopped to find something to eat, when I was interrupted by the ringing of the doorbell. When I answered the door, an American voice asked if Colin or Steffi were in. I explained that they were not, and he said that he was a neighbour and had just made a stir-fry which he wanted some help to eat. He was disappointed when I said I had eaten, but showed no surprise at finding a complete stranger in the flat. He went back to his own home saying,

"Gee! I've sure got some eating to do!"

At half-past seven, the telephone rang. It was Edna, who reported that the car had arrived as promised, that Wilf, the driver, was pleased with it, and that he would arrive as planned on the following afternoon. Harry had been to see her and assured her that everything was fine at my end and handed over the money that had been collected so far. At this point we had £1200 in the Charity account.

I pored over the map of Edinburgh, which had a scale of 1:2500, or two and a half inches to the mile. I marked the spot where the flat is and again the point that I wanted to reach. I then laid a straight-edge between the two marks in order to examine the route I should take. The first half a mile was rather complicated, it involved moving with the University on my right until I came to a green park area on my left, and then there was a right turn after about 200 yards which would bring me out onto the road out of the city that I wanted. All I needed to do then was to count the number of roads to be passed. It all seemed quite straightforward.

The next task was to leave the flat as tidy as I could. This was easier now that I had packed my kit, but tidying is not a chore that I am naturally good at. I did what I could. By this time I was ready for a drink and my bed. It occurred to me then that I had not planned what I would say to the students when I spoke to the school the next morning, but I fell asleep before I could do anything about it. Even if I had been able to make notes, I would not have been able to read them, so my speech would just have to be spontaneous.

Day Twelve

It was Thursday, 11th April. I was up early, had breakfast and stacked everything ready to go into the car by the time Charles came for me. As to the talk I was about to give; my mind was still a complete blank. The school is quite large and pleasantly situated, the students I met seemed cheerful and well-mannered and although I was nervous, everything was done to make me feel at ease. The headmaster greeted me and took us to his study where I asked how long he wanted my talk to be, and how would I know when it was time to stop. He said that after the usual assembly for prayers they would have the announcements for the day, and then there would be five minutes for me at the end. A bell would ring when assembly came to an end and this would be the signal to finish. He informed me that this assembly was only for half of the school- only about 350 students.

Only 350! it wouldn't have mattered at that point if he had said only three, I still couldn't think of a word to say.

How had I got myself into this ! Nervously I followed the Headmaster into the Hall and on to the stage. After the prayers, of which mine at least were more than usually heartfelt, members of staff made announcements concerning their various departments. Then it was my turn. The Headmaster introduced me to my unseen audience and I stood there forcing myself to say something. I wished them "Good Morning" and told them why I was doing the walk. There was no sound at all, I could have been in a room talking to myself. I needed some response from the audience. In desperation I told a joke about a blind friend of mine who after making a parachute jump for charity, was asked how he knew he was near the ground. The reply, of course, was that he felt the dog's lead go slack! Maybe it isn't very funny, but it did the trick for me, I heard a laugh, and as a result had an audience I could talk to. The bell duly rang for the end of Assembly, but the headmaster indicated that I should continue. I carried on talking for another five minutes before concluding by thanking them for their attention, and suggesting a little prayer for fine weather might be appropriate.

I was taken next to the entrance hall to meet again with the girls and the teacher that I had walked with from Queensferry. There were some photographs taken for the school magazine. We stood talking for a while, and Charles had offered to take me home, I suggested that it would help me if he could take me to the outer boundary of Edinburgh instead, so that I only had to do the walk one way. This meant, of course, that this small part of the walk would actually be done in the opposite direction from all the rest, but I couldn't see that that would make a big difference to the fact that the distance had been covered. The headmaster thought it was a very strange way of going on, but nevertheless was happy for Charles to take the time to drop me as I had requested. I took my leave, thinking that I had probably disrupted the school day quite enough. It had been quite an experience, and thanks to the help and kindness I received, an enjoyable one. I left taking a generous donation made by the school.

Charles knew the area that I wanted be, and set me down in the car park of a Public House. This was convenient as it would be easy for Wilf to stop there to drop me off on the way out. I said good-bye to Charles and felt that it was difficult to give him adequate thanks for the help he had been to me. I promised to send a postcard from Land's End and when he asked when that would be I replied,

"The last day of this month"

Why I said that I don't know, but from then on that became my self-imposed goal.

The wind was pushing at my back as I walked, making the going so easy and except for one little squall it was dry. I should have enjoyed it, but at the back of my mind was the headmaster's surprise at my unconventional way of walking this part in the wrong direction, and this, coupled with the fact that it was easy and comfortable, with none of the challenge and problems of earlier days, and I began to wonder if I should really be doing it this way. There was only one way to satisfy my conscience.

There was a cafe situated conveniently near the road where I was to turn off to the University. I stopped there for a cup of tea before setting off to retrace my footsteps. It was only eleven o'clock and I had nothing else to do. The going this way into the wind was much more difficult, and I realised how daft I was being, but at least it was honest daftness. When I reached the Pub car park, I made a ceremonial tour around it to celebrate my self-satisfaction and then set off to find a bus stop in order to get back to the Cafe. Its always a problem for me to locate a bus stop at all, never mind find out if it is the right one. There weren't many people about and those that were had usually passed me before I knew they were there, so it was difficult to ask for help. After about ten minutes, I literally walked into two people standing at the kerbside. I apologised and told them I wanted to catch a bus which would drop me somewhere near the University. As it turned out they were standing at the bus stop, and waiting for the same bus, and with the unvarying kindness that the Edinburgh folk had shown me they insisted on paying my fare, and made sure that I got off at the right place. It was now almost one o'clock, time for a drink and a sandwich in the Cafe before returning to the flat to await Wilf's arrival sometime after two o'clock.

Everything was as neat and tidy as I could make it, and time hung heavy on my hands as I waited for Wilf to arrive. I was impatient to be on my way. Now the minutes were creeping by, I was doubly pleased that I had done the morning's walk both ways, since it had taken up some time and had satisfied my conscience.

At half past two I went outside, thinking that Wilf might have difficulty finding the flat but I needn't have worried, he arrived at that moment. My impulse was to throw my things into the car and set off. However, I restrained myself and tried to consider Wilf who had driven a long way that day. He said he had eaten already, but he would like a cup of tea. While we drank our tea, Wilf admired the view, and then seemed ready to discuss plans for the day. Inside my mind was jumping up and down with impatience to be on my way, but I tried to hide it as I felt sure that Wilf needed a break. I suspect I was not very good at disguising my feelings, as after about half an hour, Wilf suggested that we set off.

It didn't take long to put the things I got ready into the car, and we were about to lock up, when I suggested as an afterthought that he had a quick look round to see if anything had been forgotten. This he did, and found not only all my spare socks piled neatly on to a chair, but also a woollen hat and a pair of gloves. Another blow to my independence!

It was half past three when we reached the car park at Eskbank, the place had already walked from and to and from again that day. I set off again, only this time it was into a gale that threatened to blow me all the way back again. I hadn't gone far when the squalls turned into driving rain. Soon my feet were soaked and when Wilf said that he had found somewhere for us to stay about a mile further on, I was pleased. That mile did not take long, and soon we were installed at the Dugan Inn at Gorebridge. I had made only about twelve or thirteen miles progress that day.

The Inn was crowded. the wind had blown down a number of trees blocking the road and bringing down telephone lines. Several drivers had lucky escapes to tell. One who had had a tree fall just in front of him, damaging his lorry, was very shaken.

It was still too early to eat, so we sat for a while in the Lounge with a drink listening to tales of near disasters in the gale. By eight o'clock there were still no telephones working and we realised that our wives would be getting increasingly worried at not hearing from us, especially since Wilf's wife, Margaret, would not even be assured of his safe arrival. There was nothing we could do.

Our dinner, when it came was well-cooked and tasty, but far more than either of us could eat, in fact, Wilf remarked that one dinner would have been enough for the two of us. As we had asked, the hotelier let us know as soon as the telephones were working again, and although this was at twenty past nine, it was some time later that we actually got near enough to the telephones to make our calls, since others had managed to get there before us. As we had guessed, Edna and Margaret had spoken to each other and had decided between them that something terrible had happened.

Although Edna was immensely relieved to hear that we were alright, she was not pleased that I had been in too much of a rush to leave Edinburgh to let them know that Wilf had arrived safely. Apparently she had tried to telephone us at the flat at about three 'o clock to tell us that a lady who lived near Gorebridge had offered us food and lodging for the night. This lady was a friend of a friend, and her home was at Stow, about ten miles south of Gorebridge. Having heard about the walk, she was anxious to help, and in fact we later discovered that she had driven out to try and find us, but the conditions had been too bad. I regretted being so full of my own thoughts that it had not occurred to me to inform Edna of Wilf's arrival. It seemed that the weather in Shropshire was apparently quite good, and it must have been impossible for her to imagine the terrible weather we were experiencing. I was happy to reassure Edna that all was well, and to apologise for the worrying time she had had.

By this time I was ready to fall into the bed which looked extremely comfortable, but first I had to study the map. Wilf was intrigued by what I was doing and asked about its significance. I recited the route as I had memorised it, telling him the distances and places and areas where there might be some difficulties. I had traced a route as far as Hawick, which was 37 miles, and suggested that as my target for the day. I did admit that I had not walked that distance on any day so far, and would be prepared to settle for a stopping place as near to that point as I could get.

I told Wilf of my practise of walking before breakfast, and he agreed to set off at 7.45 a.m. to fetch me back for my morning sustenance. I guessed that I would be about two miles from Stow by then. Wilf asked if it would bother me if he kept the light on for a while in order to read. I explained that unless the light was shining directly onto my eyes, I couldn't see it at all, and that he could read as much as he liked. There are even benefits to be found in having such limited sight on some occasions!

Day Thirteen

It was the twelfth April. At six o'clock on this cold damp morning I set off in high spirits determined to make up for what I considered to be a wasted day and a half becalmed in Edinburgh. The wind had dropped making conditions much easier than on the previous day. As I walked while one part of my mind concentrated on where I was going, another was working out all kinds of calculations. Nine miles, I thought, that's just over one per cent of the whole distance. I was always aware of exactly what proportion of the distance I had covered....it was only when I interrupted myself during a phase of this kind of lateral thinking that I realised that I had been falling headlong into a trap which must beset anyone engaged in a similar challenge. I was in danger of doing the walk for my own personal satisfaction, and of putting the fund-raising aspect into second place. I was then able to see my time in Edinburgh as a useful and contributive one, and felt that I had sorted something out.

The A71 was quiet and I made good progress along this quiet meandering road that for much of the way follows the course of the River Gala. There was occasional drizzle but it was coming from the west, and not into my face, so it was not a handicap. It was exactly eight o'clock when Wilf caught up with me. I had walked at least eight miles and had reached a point between Fountainhall and Torquhan. Wilf drove past and waited in a lay-by about a quarter of a mile further on. On the way back for breakfast Wilf said that he had been having some trouble with the windscreen wiper on the drivers' side. At the moment it was not a major problem, but in very wet conditions it could become one, so after he had returned me to the lay-by, he would go on to find a garage where he could get it fixed. Breakfast was a huge meal; Scottish appetites must be enormous. I had worked up a good appetite and thoroughly enjoyed my feast.

By this time Wilf had packed all our gear ready to go into the car, arranged for us to collect coffee and sandwiches for the day and checked the room to make sure that nothing had been left. This last action was a great help to me, since my way of doing such a check is to walk all over the floor and to feel over the bed and any shelves. I had lost a few things, socks, a toothbrush and a hat, but nothing really essential.

The car we were using was a bigger model than the hire car and we now had less gear, so not only was it easier to pack, but the things we wanted would be more accessible.

We paid our bill, ensured that the log book was signed and gratefully

72

accepted a donation before setting off for the lay-by where I was to start again on my journey south. It was not quite half past nine when I started walking. I had asked Wilf if he would find time to telephone Irene McLaughlan, the lady who had been looking out for us, to thank her and to explain that we could not accept her kind offer of accommodation since I hoped to walk another twenty three miles that day. Wilf said he would stop at the next telephone box before getting the windscreen wiper repaired.

I was very surprised when, less than an hour later, I found Wilf waiting for me in Stow with a lady by his side. Irene is a charming lady, and I was pleased to have an opportunity to thank her personally for her concern. We spoke for a while of mutual friends, took some photographs and it was time for me to be on my way again, this time heading for Selkirk. As I set off it started to rain. It was steady and continuous and although I had to wear my waterproofs which was a nuisance, there was no wind to cause any hindrance. After about two miles I came to Bowland, where I turned right over a river, I think it may still be the Gala, and onto the B710 for the next two or three miles through Clovenfords and on to Caddenfoot. Here I turned left along the A707 towards Selkirk. This road runs alongside the River Tweed for two miles before the river goes east and the road south. This was where we had arranged to meet and Wilf was waiting for me. It was by now lunch time, and I was pleased to be out of the rain for a while. My feet were still dry, but on one of my stumbles I had landed on my hands in a puddle and somehow managed to scoop water up my sleeve and wet my shirt - I don't know how I managed it ! Anyway, it was a fairly simple matter to find a dry shirt.

Wilf had found a garage which had tightened the nut on the wiper blade as they had not been able to supply a new one. This was an improvement but still not entirely satisfactory. It was a problem that we could do without.

It was two o'clock when we set out again. I was still about thirteen miles from Hawick and I was determined to be there by six o'clock so I kept up a good pace and did my best to ignore the persistent rain. Leaving the A707 south of Selkirk I turned left along the A699 for a mile before rejoining the A7. The road was much busier now and there was a lot of surface water, so once again I had the problem of spray to contend with. However it was not as bad as it had been further north when combined with fierce headwinds. There were no more diversions before Hawick so I was able to concentrate on keeping up my pace and getting there. At about four o'clock the rain eased and then stopped, but I dare not take off my waterproofs as I was still being sprayed regularly and occasionally, when me, a large puddle and an even larger lorry coincided, I had a very cold shower!

I stopped for a while near Ashkirk where I had a drink and discussed my progress with Wilf. The plan was that Wilf would stay with me until five o'clock, and then go on into Hawick to find somewhere to stay. At five o'clock I had reached Appletreehall, less than two miles from Hawick (pronounced Hoyk) and when I reached the town boundary, I had to wait a

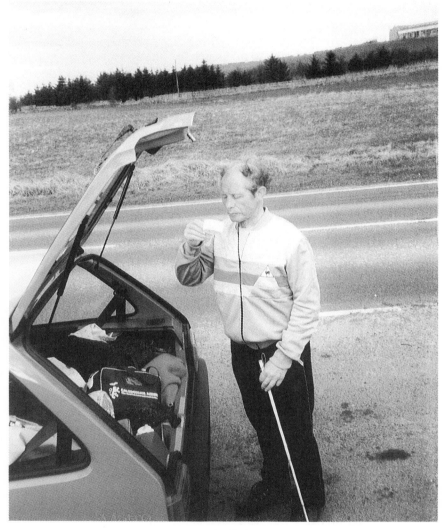

Re-fuelling

few minutes for Wilf to arrive and guide me to the Brenlands Guest house where we were to spend the night.

As I stood waiting, a lorry pulled up and the driver asked if I could direct him to Well. I had noticed this name while studying the map, so although I hadn't been there I was able to give him some help. He noticed the sweat shirt I was wearing which had been given to me along with a donation by the licensee of The Plough Inn at Wistanstow in Shropshire, and advertising their Real Ale. The driver said he had been born near there, and he was surprised that someone so far away from home was able to give him directions. He would have been even more surprised if he had realised how little I could see.

By now it was nearly six o'clock, which meant that I had been on the road for nearly twelve hours, except for meal stops, and for most of the time it had been raining heavily. I didn't even feel unduly tired and was convinced that I could have kept going if my target had not been reached. However, I was pleased to be indoors and eager for a warm bath and a change into dry clothes.

Wilf had unpacked the things that were wanted, and all I had to do was to look after myself. I emerged from the bathroom to find that my wet clothes had been hung to dry and a pot of tea had been made. Dinner was not until half past seven, so there was time to make a telephone call. Mr. Brennan, the guest house owner, offered the use of his telephone. I called Edna and asked her to ring me back in order to minimise his expense. Edna was following my progress on a map with the route and mileages marked, and duly reporting to the grandchildren who were marking their own maps with flags. It was good to know that they were so involved. It took me a little while to convince her that I wasn't utterly exhausted after walking thirty seven miles. I even called in Wilf to bear witness to the fact that I was fine. I was told that a friend of ours had a daughter who lived in Carlisle, and that she and her husband wanted us to stay in their house. I had to think about what time I would arrive.

Edna also passed on the information that the Kendal Branch of the Voluntary Society for The Blind had heard about my walk and had not only offered accommodation for a night but were also willing to help us if we wanted to do some collecting there. All this was good news, but I needed time to assimilate it and to work out a timetable. At this point I handed over the telephone to Wilf, so that he could write down the names and telephone numbers of the people we needed to contact, and I concentrated on the calculations. Wilf appeared to have complete faith in my ability to be where I said I would be at any particular time. I knew that it was forty four miles from Hawick to Carlisle and I knew that this was more than a day's walking.

Therefore I decided to think more about timing than about distances. I decided that I would walk until half past five, and then use the car to take me the remaining distance into Carlisle. This meant that we should arrive at sometime before six o'clock.

This calculation enabled Wilf to telephone our hosts in Carlisle, Roy and Jane Atkin to find out if this time would be convenient to them. They were quite happy with this, and gave us precise directions for finding their house.

The Kendal situation was much more complicated because it was still about ninety miles away. I knew that if we were to spend time collecting, it would be necessary to arrive in Kendal by three o'clock at the latest, and this meant spending the previous night not more than twenty miles north of Kendal. This would mean covering seventy miles in the next two days! I simply decided to try and do one more hour each day. Wilf accepted this, perhaps hiding any doubts he may have felt, and telephoned our helper in Kendal, arranging to meet her so that she could direct us to our overnight accommodation.

This forward planning helped me to set my targets and suited me, but it was hard on the drivers who, whether I liked it or not, felt responsible for me, and had no way of knowing whether I was pushing myself too hard or not. Wilf did point out that this plan left no margin for error if anything went wrong. I was realistic enough to know that any number of things could go wrong, a pulled muscle, blisters, or worst of all eye strain. This is something I suffer from frequently, especially after a period of concentrated effort, or of trying to see in poor light. I wake up in the night with my eyes throbbing, and the symptoms of a severe migraine. I am sometimes sick, and at least, such an attack would put me out of action for a whole day.

Edna has frequently told me that these attacks are largely self-inflicted because I have not accepted my limited vision and at times, complete blindness. I knew there was some truth in this, so I tried to avoid using my eyes to make out anything that I didn't need to see. I would close my eyes whenever possible during the evening, and only make an effort to study the route. So far I had been fortunate.

Mr. Brennan was justly proud of his cooking and we enjoyed a delicious meal that evening before a relaxed evening in the comfortable lounge. Wilf watch television and read for a while, and I studied the next day's route. I went to bed at half past ten, but for the first time since I had started off, I lay awake for some time. Unlike me, I was beginning to worry about what might go wrong - perhaps because things had gone so smoothly up to now. However, not being one to waste time in worry about things that may never happen, I slept.

Day Fourteen

The thirteenth April. Despite my restless start to the night, I was up and out by six o'clock. It was a fine morning, cold and with a light northerly breeze giving me an encouraging pat on the back the walking was easy. There was less traffic about, perhaps because it was a Saturday and I made steady progress, even benefiting from a little sunshine. However, I couldn't quite shake off the feeling that something was going to go wrong. I tried telling myself not to be silly, and to enjoy the excellent conditions and then the niggling voice in my head managed to convince me that if all was well with me, then perhaps it was my driver who was having the problems. This thought took such a hold that I almost turned back, and my relief was enormous when Wilf pipped his horn in greeting as he passed and pulled up into the next lay-by. These feelings were very strange to me as I am not normally an imaginative person nor a worrier.

The walk this morning was along the A7 through a pleasant hilly countryside and for much of the time alongside the River Teviot. After leaving Hawick I had stayed on the north side, passing Branxholme, Newmill and Broadhaugh. I had reached Teviothead by the time Wilf arrived to take me back for breakfast, a distance of nine miles. I returned to Hawick with a healthy appetite, and well pleased with my progress. Mr. Brennan had filled our flask, provided a good lunch and signed the log. Wilf did his customary check to make sure we had left nothing behind before driving me back to Teviothead. It was shortly after ten o'clock when I resumed the walk.

I was still travelling along the A7, which was undulating with high hills, or fells or pikes or whatever the local name is rising on either side of me. The Ewes Water flows alongside and as the wind was behind me and the sun was shining, I at last dismissed my unnamed worries and began to enjoy the walk. As the conditions were so favourable, I was able to appreciate the interesting landscape, especially during the periods when there was little traffic passing by. The traffic, however, became heavier as the day wore on.

From Teviothead to Ewes is nine miles and during this stretch I can only recall seeing one inhabited building, the Mosspaul Hotel. There may, of course, have been others, but I didn't see them. I stopped for lunch near Ewes, which is about twenty three miles from Carlisle.

I knew that I would not be able to cover the remaining distance on foot in the rest of the day, but nevertheless felt quite content that with another four hours walking ahead of me, I would get close enough to have only a few miles left to do the next day. I was satisfied with my progress so far and my confidence was growing.

After lunch, the walking was equally pleasant, and I was aware of some spectacular scenery. After an hour I passed through Langdale and crossed over the river which was now wider and had become, I believe, the River Esk which winds along by the road for the next twelve miles. To the east and below me the river flows through the village of Canonbie, a popular place for campers, their caravans and tents creating splashes of colour against the green backcloth of the valley.

Before setting of on the last hour and a half of the day I stopped briefly for a drink and a change of boots and socks. I had by now walked almost four hundred miles, and the Brasher boots which I had worn for most of those miles were showing real signs of wear so I thought that by changing boots more frequently I would even out the wear . I think this was also better for my feet. One snag was that by now the Hawkins boots which had been really comfortable were now a little tight, as if my feet had spread. I decided therefore to use that pair first. My third pair of boots were old friends and comfortable in any conditions, but they had been well worn before I set off and I thought that another hundred miles in them and I would be able to tell if the coin under my foot were heads or tails uppermost.

I soon passed through Netherby and mentally crossed another name off the list of places on the route. At five o'clock I was striding happily through Longtown, conscious that I had arranged to meet Wilf just two miles further on. With such thoughts in my mind, my concentration must have lapsed for a second, for my stride was interrupted, painfully, as I walked into a vehicle which had been left across the pavement with its front towards the road. My right knee came into contact with something, perhaps the car bumper, and the pain, for a moment, was excruciating. I didn't stop, but hopped, stumbled and limped along gasping for breath, not looking to see what type of vehicle it was, perhaps hoping to put the incident behind me as quickly as possible. After a little while the viciousness of the pain wore off, but my knee ached and I could not bend it.

I am no stranger to pain caused by stumbling and walking into things, and usually I am able to land lightly and minimise the discomfort, or to wait until it wears off. This time I was worried. Was this the catastrophe I had been expecting since last night? Just how serious was the injury?

It took me forty minutes to cover the last two miles, and although it was obvious that something had slowed me down, I did not want Wilf to know that I had hurt myself since he had enough to think about. I made a supreme effort to walk the last short distance to the waiting car without limping. Wilf was relieved to see me, especially since he was not used to my not arriving on time. He wondered aloud if he had travelled more than the agreed distance while looking for a convenient stopping place and I was happy to agree that this might have been so.

My mind was on my aching knee as we drove into Carlisle. Wilf followed the instructions he had been given and found the house without difficulty. Roy and Jane were waiting to welcome us, and after a cup of tea, I could scarcely wait to head to the bathroom and soak my bruised knee in warm water. As expected, the warmth eased the ache considerably and I began to feel a lot better. Nevertheless I was not able to sound quite so confident when I telephoned my report to Edna. I had originally planned to pass on the time of my arrival in Preston and give precise details for the people who were to met me in Kendal. However, I decided that I would save judgement until the following day, when I would know whether my knee would hold up or not.

I had covered thirty eight miles today. In two days it had been a total of seventy five miles. This made up for the time spent in Edinburgh and kept up my overall target of thirty miles per day. Another good day would see me handily placed for an early finish in Kendal on Monday. For the first time I had good reason to doubt that the next day would be a good one!

I spent a comfortable and relaxed hour and a half eating an excellent meal and talking about my progress. Roy and Jane were interested and asked many questions. In response to a query about the most difficult parts of the walking, I replied that it was undoubtedly making my way through towns. Roy suggested that as it was a fine evening, and if I was not too tired, he would walk with me through Carlisle which would overcome the difficult part of tomorrow's journey and add a mile to my total. I truthfully declared that I wasn't tired, but by this time, sitting in comfort, I had forgotten my damaged knee.

It was a clear, cold evening, and under any other circumstances I would have enjoyed a stroll through the town to the southern outskirts. However, every time I put weight on my knee it was quite painful, and although no-one seemed to notice that my right leg was not working properly, I was very grateful to get back to the house. The effort of trying to walk naturally after such a long day really began to tell, and I wished silently that I had had the sense to rest my knee during the evening.

Roy offered to make sure that I was at my start place by half past six the next morning. He knew the place as it was near to an area where frequently went to watch birds, which was a hobby of his. He had once worked as an R.S.P.B. Warden. Wilf was pleased as it meant he did not have to do his normal early morning run.

I sat for an hour in the cosy lounge, before heading off to my room to make sure that the next day's route was firmly absorbed, and to do anything I could to prevent my aching knee from keeping me awake. This was a fairly remote possibility, since the only medical aids I know about are either a sticking plaster or an aspirin! I hunted in the first aid kit, and found a bottle of something that smelled like liniment of some kind. I had no idea whether it would help, but rubbed it in to the damaged part in the hope that it might. In fact I had no problems going straight to sleep, staying awake only long enough to wonder how I might explain the rather strong smell the following morning.

Day Fifteen

Roy woke me at ten to six with a cup of tea. I was in a deep sleep and for a moment or two I didn't know where I was. This was most unusual for me, for although I had brought with me my talking clock which has an alarm I had not needed it since I was awake in good time every morning. I wonder how long I might have slept on without my "alarm call" and welcome cup of tea.

I was quite practised at getting up and dressed in the dark and I laid out my clothes in order at night so that the process could be quick and quiet. It generally worked quite well, except for the odd occasion when I was discovered to be wearing something back to front. By ten past six we were out of the house and on our way to the point two miles south of Longtown where I had so gratefully finished my previous day.

Roy went off to inspect the marshy pool nearby, and told me that unless anything very interesting ornithologically were occurring, he would see me back at the house for breakfast at half past eight. He set off carrying his haversack containing binoculars and camera and also his sketch pad.

I set off a little apprehensively on that Sunday morning which was warmer than I had come to expect and fine after a wet night. My knee still ached but I decided that the best plan was to forget about it and carry on as if nothing were wrong. I stepped out and as the light improved and the cool clear air invigorated me I found myself singing as I made my way along an almost deserted road. The A7 was a fitting audience for my tuneless but cheerful song, since I have learned to my cost that whenever I break out into spontaneous song the response from any human audience is without exception scathing. Maybe I am short on musical talent, but I was so pleased that my knee, although a little stiff and aching was carrying me along alright and did not seem to have sustained any serious or permanent harm that I am sure I could be forgiven a little musical exuberance.

I passed through the village of Blackford, which was so deserted that its entire population must have been enjoying a lie in on this April Sunday morning. Next I came to the junction where the A7 and the A74 meet at the northern end of the M6 motorway. Using the method I had practised so long ago on the A49, I safely negotiated the junction and its maelstrom of traffic which was something of a shock after the quiet roads I had just come along. I was soon back in Carlisle and more than ready for breakfast. Shortly after I arrived Roy returned and we all four enjoyed the breakfast that Jane had prepared. I enjoyed the company, and in fact spent longer there than I should, for it was half past nine by the time I left. Wilf had collected together our possessions, including freshly washed and ironed clothes thanks to Jane's efforts. My gratitude for the help and support of Roy and Jane is enormous. Not only did they make sure that we were provided with a good lunch for the day ahead, but they had also each been fund-raising at their places of work; Roy is a schoolteacher and Jane is an analyst for a water company. We went on our way therefore with their good wishes and a generous donation to the Fight for Sight. The impression that they had created that we were doing them a favour in staying with them made me feel humble, not for the first time, at this generous and unconditional help from people who thought nothing of the personal inconvenience and were pleased to offer support.

Leaving Carlisle, I set off towards the south down the old Roman road that we know as the A6. This road was to take me the estimated forty four miles through Penrith and over Shap to Kendal. Today the sun was very bright, and instead of being grateful, I was disturbed by its shining into my face. The glare was as much of a nuisance as poor light. I had anticipated that this might be a problem, and I had experimented in the past with spectacles that adjust and darken according to the brightness of the sun. However I had decided not to use them since I found that my eyes took such a long period to adjust to light changes that if I stepped into shade, it was stepping into total blackness.

After half an hour I passed under junction 42 of the M6 and was pleased to note that most of the traffic had gone onto the motorway leaving me in relative peace away from the constant noise. The road was straight, but not quite as straight as it looks on the map. I felt refreshed and able to enjoy the clean air around me and the open countryside. I had good memories of walking in this area in previous years and knew that I was in the sort of land where I felt most at home. What it lacked in beauty and variety, the elements of the Shropshire landscape that I love, it made up for in grandeur and I could feel the challenge of each surrounding peak inviting me to discover the view from its topmost point. I mentally responded to the challenge, eager to return someday and explore the delights of the place, but knowing sadly that if it were to happen, it could only be done if someone would agree to accompany me. Such thoughts made me only too aware of my limitations, and helped me to pull myself out of my drifting, dreaming mood, and concentrate on covering another twenty miles that day.

Relishing the atmosphere and the pleasant Spring weather, I pushed on, through Low Hesketh, then High Hesketh. On my right beyond the valley of the River Petteril the traffic rumbled north and south on the motorway in another world. The lunch time stop was at Plumpton, famous for its

Racecourse. I could see splashes of yellow blue and white on the green canvas below me, and realised I was looking at another caravan site. Half an hour was long enough for lunch and a change of boots and I was ready to set off again for Plumpton Head and Penrith.

During the stop, Wilf surprised me by asking if I thought the liniment had been any help to my injured knee. My attempt to fool him had clearly been futile. I answered truthfully that the liniment had helped, and quickly changed the subject. By now my knee was aching and felt a little swollen, but it was still bearing me up with no real difficulty, and I didn't want to make anything of it, being certain that another night's rest would put it right. I certainly didn't want Wilf to worry about it.

After Penrith the road goes through Eamont Bridge, Clifton, Lowther and Hackthorpe, staying alongside the motorway for about six miles. I wove in and out, crossing over it twice and under it once in a very short distance. At Hackthorpe I met up with Wilf who suggested that as we were only twenty miles from Kendal, he would go on and find somewhere for us to stay for the night. I didn't want to go off the road although there were a couple of inviting villages not far away. I asked Wilf to find somewhere, if possible, that I could set off from in the morning without wasting time getting back on the right road. Once. earlier, I had walked a quarter of a mile up a hill just to get back on the route, and although it was no problem physically, I had not liked amount of useful time it had taken up, and spent much of the day thinking, "I would have been that much further ahead by now!"

I had just crossed under the motorway again when I saw Wilf next. He had found the King's Arms in Shap which was just a mile down the road. I reckoned that Shap was only about fourteen miles from Kendal, and was therefore an ideal place to stop. My knee was beginning to be a problem, and I was pleased to reach the King's Arms. From the place where the A6 goes under the M6 the roads diverge on their route southwards and it is some distance before they come together again, so that at Shap they are about half a mile apart, and far enough away for the continuous hum of traffic not to bother us.

The King's Arms is a comfortable traditional Inn. A friendly, no-nonsense sort of place with clean, warm rooms. We had an en suite bathroom with a lovely, deep bath sometimes condemned as uneconomic but to me a real luxury. It must have become apparent by now how much I had come to value a soak in the tub at the end of each day's walking. This time I also wanted to examine my knee in privacy without drawing Wilf's attention to it.

It is only possible for me to see my knees when my legs are at right angles to my body. A detailed examination showed some swelling, but I had worried that it might be worse. I was reasonably satisfied that a good rest overnight and a relatively easy day to follow should just about put it right.

While Wilf was having his turn in the bathroom, I rechecked the distance between Kendal and Shrewsbury and tried to work out where I would need to be by the end of each day if I was to reach Shrewsbury by the end of Friday's walk. The route passed through several towns, and this was where I knew I might encounter problems. Some towns seemed to have a fairly direct road through, but others seemed to be indecipherable mazes. It was pointless worrying about what I didn't know, so I decided to work it out on distances. I had a few names of places in my mind, and felt a little more in control. When I told Wilf what I had been up to, he suggested that instead of using the actual places as targets, I should think in terms of "to the north or south of ..." which would give me more tolerance, and the opportunity to make up for a bad day with a good one. I liked this idea, and when I telephoned Edna I told her that I would be in Kendal the following day as I had promised. On Tuesday, I would be near Preston, on Wednesday, north of Warrington, on Thursday, south of Warrington and on Friday, if my luck held, would see me in Shrewsbury.

Edna could scarcely believe that I should be there so soon. She was happy to have the information, as it meant that she could go ahead and organise accommodation where it had been offered and make arrangements for the next change of driver. I think it must have seemed that after being so far away, I was now within reach of home and I think it made her feel more comfortable about the rest of the walk.

Her news was that the caravanette had been repaired and that my son had taken care of the cost as another contribution to the cause. She was also very pleased with the way in which funds were coming in and being promised. She estimated that I might raise about £4,000. Apparently the kitchen at home resembled an office with the telephone, typewriter and trays of papers all over our large scrubbed wooden kitchen table. Every post brought donations, and even on that Sunday, an envelope containing £10 had been put through the door. The charity organisers thought my driver should have a car phone and were trying to arrange it, though I was not sure how useful it might be. However, I was heartened by the fact that my efforts really seemed to be raising money and that there were no major problems.

There was some time to wait before we had our meal, so we had a drink, and listened to the light hearted banter that was going on between the barman and two of his customers. The barman had asked about what I was doing when we booked in, and he had asked for a collecting tin. His attempts to persuade 'voluntary' contributions from his other customers aroused many friendly insults, but nevertheless everyone there was exceedingly generous. We talked later with a woman who worked there, and met her father, who suffered from Retinitis Pigmentosa, but in his case it was a strain that is carried by the women who are often not badly affected, and passed to their sons, who often lose their sight completely. My type of the disease is not so intrusive in the family, and just crops up occasionally. This family in Shap had many members affected by the disease, and perhaps the fact that in this happy friendly pub everyone knew them may explain the generosity we encountered there. I'm sure that the cost of the excellent dinner was unusually cheap as well.

At ten o'clock I went to the bedroom. I felt that it had been a long day, and I wanted to start early, as usual. I studied my route, and applied more liniment to my knee. None of this took long, it was a short distance to Kendal and there were no difficulties that I could foresee.

Day Sixteen

Monday, fifteenth of April. A glorious morning, very clear and just cold enough for me to feel a nip to the nose and fingers and to encourage me to get a move on. At five forty five I was on my way on the long almost continuous downhill from Shap towards Kendal. Poetic I am not, but on such a morning I understand anyone feeling;

"Oh! to be in England, now that spring is here"

During the first hour there was hardly any traffic and although it built up a little after that, it was still reasonably quiet. The sun rose on my left far beyond the motorway, a great bright ball that I dare not look at. The downhill walking was so easy that I was almost running. The road was dry and clean and the countryside open blemished only by the quarries that seem a must to most hilly or mountainous areas.

There are no villages on this stretch of road and only the occasional dwelling. I crossed several small bubbling rivers including the Birk Beck and the Borrow Beck as they tumble off Shap fell and down into the dales. Wilf caught up with me at Watchgate, within four miles of Kendal and on the way back for breakfast we discussed how to make the most of the spare time we would have. As usual, I wanted to go on and cover more of the distance, but Wilf, in his common-sense way suggested that it might be as well for us to take our time over breakfast and then for me to do two hours walking which would take me well beyond Kendal. Then we could have a break and freshen up before meeting the people who had offered to help with collecting. This plan seemed reasonable to me particularly as I was still concerned about my knee which, though it hadn't interfered with my walking, felt swollen and bruised.

Breakfast was the leisurely affair we had promised ourselves and it was after ten o'clock when we got on our way again. Indulging in luxury though we were, the other party of walkers in the hotel, who were doing Wainwright's Coast to Coast Walk, and who were marking the half way point at Shap took even longer than us and didn't seem in a great hurry to get on with the second half. Wilf laughed when I commented on this, saying that it wasn't them who were tardy, but me who always had to be on the move.

The barman presented us with a heavy collecting tin and wished us well and we promised to send him a card from Land's End. I thought it took a long time to get to the point where I was to resume my walk, and Wilf pointed out that I had covered ten miles before breakfast that morning.

By now it was considerably warmer, the sun shone from a clear blue sky and a gentle northerly breeze patted me encouragingly on the back. If I could have planned the weather, then this was what I would have organised, this and the time to appreciate it. Wilf was to walk through Kendal with me, so after dropping me off he drove away to find somewhere to park, and I had walked through Meal Bank and reached the outskirts of the town when we met again.

Wilf had parked on the south side of the towns so we strolled through the centre, stopping to look in shop windows occasionally, and I was on the look out for a good spot to collect. I like a place where you can be seen easily, where the pavement narrows, and where there is a steady stream of passers-by, but not a torrent. It was unusual for me to have time to look around me.

When we reached the car it was after twelve and I decided to go on for about three miles before finishing for the day. Wilf and I met up again at a place near where the A6 crosses the River Kent. We found a grassy bank and enjoyed a pic-nic in the sunshine, a real luxury. An hour later we returned by car to the car park, packed our collecting gear in a rucksack and walked back into the centre of Kendal. The collecting equipment consisted of tins, stickers and huge eye-catching T-shirts, big enough to wear over a sweater. The motif on the T-shirts was the one used by the Fight for Sight Campaign, with the silhouette of the head of a blindfolded child. I didn't mind wearing such a conspicuous shirt, especially since it was designed to allow warm clothing underneath. It can be cold work, standing on one spot for a number of hours.

In Kendal, we found a suitable spot and began to collect. A few minutes after this, the two ladies who had said they would meet us there arrived and introduced themselves. They each took a tin and went off to find a suitable spot to collect. There were not many people about, but those who passed by gave generously. Our two helpers left before four as they had children at school, but not before handing over two heavy tins and a personal donation. Wilf and I stayed on until five o'clock, before returning to the car and setting out to find our lodgings. Later, when we counted up, two and a half hours collecting from us, and invaluable help from the two ladies had raised a total of over £130.

It took us a while to find the house where we were to stay. I think we did a left turn instead of a right or vice versa, and of course, I'm no help at all with looking for road names. Eventually we found it, a pleasant suburban house where we were welcomed and made to feel instantly comfortable by our hosts, the Reverend and Mrs. Mason. After a cup of tea we were shown to a comfortable bedroom, and asked to join the couple for dinner in about half an hour. Mrs. Mason apologised for the early dinner, explaining that they had a Bible class later that evening. The meal was one of the best of the many good meals we had on our journey and we had scarcely left the table and made our way into the sitting room, before people began arriving for the Bible Class. The telephone rang and the Reverend Mason answered it. He said that it was a lady with a Midland's accent asking for me. It was Edna, a bit mystified by being identified as having a Midland's accent since she had been born and spent much of her early life in Yorkshire. As usual, she had everything well organised and all our prospective hosts had been informed of our progress and told when we expected to be in their area. She had also had an offer from a cousin of Harry Field who lived in Preston, to meet me on the north side of the town and walk with me to the southern outskirts. I was pleased to accept the offer since it would not only save time and considerable map study, but it would also be easier on my driver.

The telephone rang again almost immediately, and this time it was someone who said that they knew me and could they come along to see me. I spent the next few minutes waiting for this arrival wondering who it might be! Since Edna does all the writing in our house, I scarcely ever know anyone's address.

When they arrived I was pleased to greet a friend I had known for many years. Her first husband and I were in the A.T.C. together in 1941 and then from 1953 we had been near neighbours for over thirty years until after his death, when she had moved to be near her daughter who lives in Kendal. She had recently remarried and it was her new husband who brought Joan and her daughter, Gillian to meet me. They had seen a report in the local newspaper about my walk and had found my address by contacting the newspaper. Their company was a real delight and both Wilf and I were sorry when they left after about an hour and a half. They would not leave before making a generous donation, wishing me well, and issuing an invitation for the future, if we should return to this beautiful part of the country.

By this time the Bible Class had finished and we met its members, the Mason's brought us all coffee and the evening continued, the noise and chatter getting less as they gradually left and by half past nine, there were just the four of us. The Reverend Mason gave us a donation from the Bible Class. It seemed that all I did was take. I wished that there was something more I could do or say to all the kind, helpful and generous people to express my thanks. I could only say "Thank you very much" which seemed so inadequate to express my heartfelt appreciation.

My referring to Ian and Irene Mason as the Reverend Mason and his wife may have given the impression of a formal evening, in fact it was the opposite. They made us feel very much at home, and in fact it was Wilf who suggested that we say Grace before dinner, and I think that went out of their way to make sure that we did not feel uncomfortable.

It was after eleven o'clock when I excused myself and retired to the bedroom. It had been a good and interesting day, but nevertheless it had been quite wearing, and I was very tired. I found it hard to assimilate my route for the next day, and while I was trying to study it, my eyes kept closing. Rather than risk straining my eyes I decided to break my own rule, and leave it until the morning. On this occasion, I was not planning to leave before breakfast. The Masons were early risers and with a bit of luck we should be on our way by eight o'clock the next morning.

Day Seventeen

Having been provided with a good breakfast and more than enough sandwiches and coffee to last the day, we said our good-byes to the couple who had made us feel so welcome. They wished us a safe journey and presented yet another donation, this time from themselves. It was eight o'clock in the morning, Tuesday, 16th April. The weather was a continuation of the conditions of the day before, except that the northerly breeze was a little stronger and its pat on the back was on occasion quite a strong push - any help was welcome!

As I left the point we had reached the day before, I was conscious that for the first time since leaving John O'Groats I had not got the route for the day clearly in my mind. I had tried to look at it that morning and had the main places in the correct order, but my usual mental picture of the number, position and distance of side roads, roundabouts, turnings and intersections was missing. It was an uncomfortable feeling.

I was surprised when I passed Wilf parked in a Lay-by a little way before the road crossed over the M6 motorway after only three miles into the day's programme. He had taken everything out of the boot and was repacking it. We had been anxious to set off as early as possible, and obviously hadn't packed the car to his satisfaction. We acknowledged each other, but I didn't stop. I crossed over the motorway and continued on.

Something felt wrong! The motorway noise was growing less and it shouldn't have. I thought I remembered that road ran near to the motorway and crossed it again just north of Carnforth. I decided to carry on until I came to the next lay-by in the hope that there might be someone there who could direct me. I reached the village of Lupton, there was an empty lay-by and a sign post to Kirby Lonsdale. Although there were dozens of people passing me in cars, there was no-one to ask, so reluctantly I crossed the road and began to retrace my steps. After walking for a few minutes, I came to a lane that led in a westerly direction and thinking that this must take me towards the motorway and south of where I had crossed it, I decided to follow it. Though I was not unduly worried for myself I was concerned for Wilf, who would have no idea where I was. For that matter neither did I!

Half a mile later at a cross-roads I found a signpost pointing to the left and on it the magic word 'Carnforth' . I could have cheered, until I recalled that I was still in the lanes and still without Wilf. Relief was not far away, for ten minutes later as I passed through the village of Farleton and was walking towards the A6070, I heard a familiar voice, and Wilf was beside me. He had looked at the map and guessed what had happened, and knowing that I would not panic, had judged that he might find me at this junction. All was well.

This roundabout walking , however, had taken me an hour, and I had only progressed one mile from the point where I had spotted Wilf repacking the car. This meant that it had taken an hour and three quarters to cover four miles. It was not enough. Nevertheless a drink and a ten minute break to recount our adventures was called for. When I set off again, I was pleased to note that the road did indeed follow alongside the motorway going through Burton in Kendal before crossing it a mile north of Carnforth.

I was travelling well now. The weather was as near perfect for walking south as it could be. After Carnforth the road edges west along the coast. I could smell the sea, but I could not see it from this road which passes through Bolton-le-Sands and on towards Lancaster. I met Wilf and we stopped for lunch near Morecambe, about a mile and a half north of Lancaster. I was pleased at my progress since I had made up some of the time I had lost. The fine weather made it possible to wear my lightest boots and trainers and such small things seemed to make a difference to the ease and speed of travelling.

During the short lunch break, we discussed where we might stay that evening. I knew that some friends in Accrington had invited us to stay with them, but I calculated that I would be fifteen miles north of Accrington at the end of the day. Wilf saw no problem, saying that if he telephoned for directions, he could get us there in half an hour. I worked out where I thought I would be at half past five, the time I planned to finish on that day. My objective was a place called Catteral, a mile south of Garstang. I usually took a half hour break for lunch, but on this day I was eager to make up for lost time, and set off again after twenty minutes. In retrospect, I know that ten minutes here or there made no real difference, but then my mind was programmed to certain goals, and I tried hard to keep to the formulae.

At Lancaster, Wilf parked the car and walked with me through the town to the southern outskirts. He seemed reluctant to return to the car, it was such a pleasant day and he clearly enjoyed the chance to stretch his legs.

On the A6 the miles slipped away, through Galgate and Scorton and I was near Garstang when I next saw Wilf. He had been trying to contact Ray and Delys Ashton, our prospective hosts with no success so far. He was going to drive on to find a telephone box near to where I planned to stop walking and try again. If there was still no reply, we would have to find somewhere else to stay.

We met again at exactly half past five in the spot we had marked on the map. Wilf was smiling. He had spoken to Ray, who was going to come out and lead us back to his home. He thought this would be simpler than trying to give directions and leaving us to find the way ourselves. We still had some coffee left, and although it was now cooler, it was quite pleasant and no hardship to wait for the twenty minutes it took Ray to reach us.

A mile or so before we had stopped there had been some roadworks and I had walked into a triangular warning sign. There had been no damage done, but it reminded me of the problem I had had with my knee, and I realised that I had forgotten it completely and that it must be as good as ever.

Ray and Delys have been friends for a long time, but we hadn't met for some while, and we had a great deal to talk about. I sat in the car with Ray as he drove to Accrington. He took a roundabout route, and pointed out places of interest and local beauty spots. Unfortunately, I find it difficult to appreciate scenery while travelling by car as we have usually passed it before I have had chance to find it. Wilf followed us to the house.

When we arrived there was a note from Delys apologising for her absence and explaining that she had to attend a meeting. There was, however, a meal prepared, and Ray was all set to look after us. There was just time for a bath and a change of clothes before the meal would be ready. It is a comfortable, modern family home, and very spacious now the children have grown up and have homes and families of their own.

After half an hour, we presented ourselves downstairs, where Ray served a delicious starter followed by an even more appetising meal. Ray is a self-employed carpenter and cabinet maker and the house contained several examples of the high quality of his work. He is no mean cook either! My offer of assistance with the clearing up after dinner was declined and it was suggested that I do my telephoning. I think most people value their china more than they do my help.

The telephone rang before I had chance to make my call. Edna had anticipated our safe arrival. She had been in contact with the couple who had offered us accommodation in the Warrington area and they had said that they would be happy for us to stay two nights with them. This was good. If our luck held it meant no further accommodation problems for the next five nights, since I intended to spend Friday, Saturday and Sunday nights at my own home. At my request, Edna had arranged for us to spend some time collecting in Shrewsbury on Saturday and she and two friends were to come along and help. Also, she had obtained permission to collect at Harry Tuffin's supermarket in Craven Arms. It was the manager of this supermarket who had so generously provided supplies at the outset of the venture.

Delys returned at around nine o'clock and after welcoming us, offered to wash our clothes and promised they would be ready by the next morning. She was as good as her word, and they were in a neat pile, washed and pressed all ready for us in the morning. I reluctantly left the cosy room at half past ten, for although I was enjoying the cheerful company, I was anxious to absorb tomorrow's route before I got too tired.. There was a considerable amount of complicated walking to do and I didn't want to get lost again.

Day Eighteen

We were up early the next morning and were given a large cooked breakfast including some of the black pudding for which this part of the country is well known. With our flask filled and enough packed food to last several days, we set off. It was eight o'clock. Ray was taking Delys to work and then he had offered to lead us back to our starting point. This suited me, since it can be difficult finding your way on a suburban housing estate and I was all for saving trouble. By nine o'clock I was at the right place and ready to set off again, it only remained to thank our host for the welcome we had received and the way in which they had cared for us.

The weather was colder, but still dry and that friendly little breeze was still behind me. Wilf stayed behind to do some telephoning and when I next saw him he explained that he had arranged for Les Jones, the man who had offered to walk with me through Preston to meet us about six miles on from our starting point at half past ten. By this time I was between Bilsborrow and Barton and only three miles from the proposed meeting point. It occurred to me that we hadn't given him much notice. Nevertheless, just as I approached the island where the M55 goes over the A6 a man pushing a bicycle came up to me and introduced himself as Les Jones. He was most apologetic that as his wife wasn't well he had not been able to offer accommodation, but in fact his contribution was very helpful to me. Pushing his bicycle with one hand, and using the other to steady and guide me, he walked for the next five or six miles through the centre of Preston and on to Bamber Bridge where Wilf was waiting for us. Having made sure that we knew our way from there, he shook hands, wished us luck and rode off on his bicycle, waving aside my thanks and saying that it had been a pleasure. His pleasure had saved me a lot of time and concern.

Half an hour later, near Leyland at a quiet roadside spot we met up for lunch. It was then we realised how much food was in the bag which Delys had given us. Not only were there enough sandwiches to last until we got home, but also a pork pie, crisps tomatoes, chocolate rolls and fruit. It was good to have such a rich source of 'fuel' to help me on my way.

This was the section of the walk that most bothered me. So much of it was through built up areas. Although I have spent most of my life in Birmingham, I now feel almost claustrophobic when there are buildings all around me. Getting through Preston so well was a weight off my mind, but there was still Wigan and Warrington to negotiate. I was now on the A49 with the M6 motorway I had just crossed to the east. The next seven miles from Clayton-le-Woods to Wigan was through fairly open country and quite straightforward for me so Wilf felt confident to drive on when we restarted after lunch and arranged to meet me at Marylebone on the north side of Wigan.

Two hours later we met as planned. The walk had been uneventful, but not as open as I had thought. Standish had turned out to be a larger place than I expected, with the A49 going through about a mile and a half of built up surroundings. It was here that I came across a lady with a dog which was standing in my way and barking madly as if to fend off intruders into his territory. The lady pulled the dog out of my way and apologised for his behaviour, saying that he was getting on in years and was going blind. I saw the parallel with myself and remarked that I knew how he felt! The lady added that the dog was getting to be a nuisance and she was afraid that she would have to have him put down. At this point my identification with the dog ended abruptly, and I hurriedly said good-bye and walked off a little faster than my usual pace.

Wilf was waiting for me. He had parked the car at Ince in Makerfield on the south side of the town and walked back to meet me. With his help and foreknowledge it didn't seem a difficult town to get through and soon we reached the place where he had left the car. A quick drink and we were off again; me to do another hour of walking and Wilf to find a telephone so that he could find out how to reach the house we were to stay that evening. We were to go to the home of David and Maira Sellers. David is my daughter-in-laws' brother, and he and his wife had been among the first to offer help and accommodation.

Much of this stretch of the walk is built up, through Abram and Golborne but it is leafy and not congested with traffic. After four miles I met up again with Wilf who was waiting in a lay-by. It was half past five and considering the type of walking that had been involved, I felt pleased with my progress, and was relieved to be still on schedule.

It was a drive of about ten miles to Sale, and Wilf following instructions from our hosts, found the house without any difficulty. David, Maira and their daughter Sarah were waiting to greet us when we arrived and soon we were installed in their large comfortable house and soon felt quite at home. After a bath and change of clothes we were ready for the meal which Maira had prepared. Once again it was a super meal, there was no doubt that I could easily become accustomed to the Gourmet fare that our hosts were providing. I made a mental note to suggest to Edna that this was the way I would like to eat from now on. I won't go into detail about her response to this suggestion!

In spite of the fact that we had been informed that some people would be coming to the house for a meeting, the meal was a pleasant, leisurely affair, and we were drinking coffee in the sitting room when the first of the ladies arrived for the meeting. Shortly after this the telephone rang, and I realised that I had been so busy eating, drinking and chatting that I hadn't found time to telephone Edna. She had telephoned, worried because she had heard nothing from me. However, she was so relieved to hear that all was well that she forgot to be cross about my forgetting to call her before this. I told her that we had accepted the offer of returning here for another night after the following day's walk, and that I hoped to reach Shrewsbury on the day after. Edna informed me that both the Shrewsbury Lions and The Shropshire Voluntary Society for The Blind had cheques to present to me and that they would be waiting in the car park of a hotel in north Shrewsbury at five o'clock on Friday. This was a pressure that I didn't want. My own deadlines were in my mind and could be adjusted, but this deadline was a fact, and I didn't want to let down these generous people, or even keep them waiting. I was sixty miles away still, and there was still the hazards of walking through Warrington and Whitchurch, though the latter didn't look too much of a problem. I was a little afraid that we were taking our good fortune for granted, and that something was sure to go wrong soon.

There was no profit in anticipating something that I hoped would never happen and Edna was doing an excellent job of organising rendezvous on the basis of my guesswork, so I did not express any concern. The doubt must have been apparent in my tone of voice, for Edna asked anxiously if these arrangements were alright. I answered truthfully that I would do my best to ensure that they were. It did mean that I should have to alter my proposed route a little. I had intended to go from Whitchurch to Shrewsbury along the quieter B5476 through Wem but as the meeting place was on the A49 it would now be best to stay on that road. The distance was the same on both routes.

The telephoning done, I returned to the sitting room for what I thought would be a quiet hour or two but it didn't work out that way. First it was three of my grandchildren who had learned that I was now at their Uncle David's house and were eager to talk to me on the telephone. This was a pleasure for me, even though it meant saying things three times to each of them in turn! Then Maira brought me a donation from the ladies at the meeting, and I asked if I could thank them. I went in and thanked them and told them a little about the walk which only took a few minutes, but then they began asking questions and their meeting almost turned into my meeting. By the time I left them, it was almost time for bed. However, I did spend a quiet hour with the family before going up to study my route and get some sleep at about eleven o'clock.

Day Nineteen

Thursday the eighteenth April. I don't think David or Maira are normally early risers, but on this occasion they brought us tea at half past six, and by half past seven we had eaten a large cooked breakfast and were on our way.

It was not a good morning as far as the weather was concerned. It was dark, cold and pouring with rain. The ride back to the starting point should have been uncomplicated, along the M63 north until we reached the M62 then west for eight miles to the M6 where we turn north for another three miles to Golborne. It sounds simple enough, but as soon as we turned on to the M63 we were in a traffic jam, stopping and starting and inching our way along. Wilf suggested that as we needed petrol it might be a good idea to leave the motorway at the next junction to find a petrol station and maybe in the meantime the traffic congestion would ease. This we did.

There was no petrol station near the exit, so we drove on until we came to one. It seemed to take ages but eventually we had filled up with petrol and returned to the motorway where the traffic was moving more freely. However after half a mile we were back in a jam. All this time it had been raining heavily, and Wilf put the windscreen wipers on to fast wipe. This was a mistake. The wiper on the driver's side stopped working altogether. All the way to the next exit we crawled along in a traffic queue moving one car's length at a time and with Wilf trying to see out through the space cleared by the passenger's wiper. I could be of no help, since I can see nothing through a curtain of rain.

The next exit, when it came, was a great relief and we set off to find somewhere where we could get the wiper repaired. Once again it seemed that we had to drive for miles before we found a garage, it probably seemed further because of the very slow pace at which we travelled. Wilf remained completely calm and appeared in control but I am sure that he was pleased when we stopped safely in the forecourt of a petrol station. He went to see if someone could help us to get the wiper fixed. Unfortunately, there were no repair facilities here, and neither did they sell spare wipers, so Wilf bought a set of spanners in the hope that we could repair it ourselves.

When we tried to tighten the wiper arm the cause of the trouble became clear; the boss at the base of the arm was split and the more we tightened it the wider the split grew. With the help of some tape and a little uncomplimentary language, we managed to reassemble it and it seemed quite secure. By now feeling wet and uncomfortable we set off again. It soon became apparent that the wiper wasn't clearing the screen properly, so into the rain we went again for another try at putting it right. This time it was more successful. A little less tape underneath and a little more on the top and the pressure was about right.

The next problem we had to solve was how to get back to the motorway. We were completely lost. Neither of us had taken much notice of the way we had come. We returned to the garage where we asked a young woman if she could direct us, but she hadn't a clue. Her very helplessness gave us a much needed laugh and reduced our tension. We set off back in the general direction from which we had come. By this time the rain was easing, and we found our way to the motorway, joining it at the next junction along from the one where we had left. The rain stopped, there was no further problem with traffic, and at last we reached the starting point.

Throughout the whole episode, Wilf had stayed calm and unruffled, and although I had been fretting inwardly at the wasted walking time, I was determined not to do or say anything that might put any more pressure on him. The result was that we had been able to see humour in the situation and put the whole thing down to experience.

It was ten o'clock and I wanted to get straight off but Wilf insisted that I have a warm drink first and put on dry boots and socks as he had done. I followed his sensible advice and was in good heart when I set off, intent on getting on as far and as fast as I could in what was left of the day. By now the walking conditions were good for me; high, light clouds, no glare and a cross wind that was more help than hindrance. Even after all that rain, the road seemed remarkably dry and although there was some spray from passing vehicles, it was not enough to bother me as I pushed myself to my best possible speed.

When I had studied the road through Warrington on my map it had seemed fairly straightforward and I didn't think it would be much trouble so I suggested to Wilf that he should go off and try and get the wiper repaired properly. He could then meet me at Stretton which is three miles south of Warrington and where the A49 crosses the M56. Wilf was not happy about this idea but I was pleased when he reluctantly agreed. I felt that he needed a break, that morning must have been very wearing for him. He stayed with me until he had seen me safely past the M62 junction and on the road into the town. As I had anticipated, I had no real trouble, though I did have to make a short diversion to find a toilet. This had been a problem for me before, as I have already explained, but at least in the countryside there was usually a convenient tree or hedge to duck behind. In a town it meant asking to be directed. In this case I asked a policeman who first of all gave me directions, and then, realising that I couldn't see very well, guided me across the road and walked with me the short distance to the nearest public convenience. I permitted myself a smile at the thought of Wilf's reaction if he had happened to see me being escorted by a policeman. He would have been convinced that I was being run in for some misdemeanour.

When I did see Wilf however, all was well. He had taken the car to a garage where they had fitted a new wiper and wiper arm. They had charged him only for the parts, and then put half into his collecting tin.

We crossed the M56 and had our lunch in the first lay-by. It was a very short break for me, for I knew that I still had a long distance to cover that day. Fortunately, the going was now easy. A good, reasonably flat road through pleasant well-managed farmland. The landscape was a little too organised and had too few hills for my taste, but it was ideal for the job I was doing. Although the road was quite busy, the traffic did not bother me.

The first seven miles of this stretch of the A49 twisted and turned through Weaverham and wove its way into Cuddington. Then the road straightened out for three miles into Cotebrook. A quarter of a mile on, and I decided to take a lane on the left to Eaton. This lane bypassed Tarporley and was a little shorter in distance. For a blessed two miles I was without the traffic, and for the space of half an hour I was able to relax my constant vigilance and concentration. This was such a relief after the inexorable whoosh! whoosh! of vehicles passing, sometimes within inches of me. One inconsiderate bramble did manage to reach out and scratch my face. I was used to this happening regularly while walking in the lanes around my home, and the absence of such attacks was one of the benefits of main road walking.

Wilf was waiting for me as I turned once again onto the A49 and was shocked and upset by my appearance. In wiping the blood from my scratched face, I had managed to spread it liberally, and according to Wilf, I looked as if I had been in a road accident. When he had recovered, and cleaned me up he asked me what time I proposed to finish walking as he wanted to let David and Maira know what time we would get back to their house. I told him that I hoped to reach Spurstow which was two or three miles further on. Wilf went off agreeing to meet me there. It was by now a quarter past five. I crossed the Shropshire Union Canal at Tiverton, and wondered how many days it would be until I came to the next Tiverton on my route, in Devon.

At ten minutes before six o'clock I reached Spurstow where Wilf was waiting. I had covered twenty nine miles which, considering the start to the day, was very satisfactory. It had been a long stint, and it felt like it. The two and a half hours of delay and difficulties that morning had been far more wearing for me than walking for the equivalent time would have been. However, I had reached the place that I had selected as my minimum target for the day, and I was now only thirty miles from Shrewsbury. The largest place I still had to go through was Whitchurch, and I knew my way through there, so despite being more tired than I had been at the end of any day's walking, I was , I'm afraid, not very quietly confident. My mood amused Wilf, as I am rarely excitable and he remarked that it was the first time I had 'bubbled' like this and talked about walking thirty miles before five o'clock as if it were a formality. Truthfully, at this point I thought it was.

The journey back to Sale was uneventful and took us about half an hour. David and Maira were dining out that evening, but Sarah provided us with a splendid meal. Whether she had prepared it I couldn't say, but she was a perfect hostess and very good and interesting company. At the time I write this, Sarah is a student at Birmingham University.

After my customary bath and change of clothes, I telephoned Edna for my regular report. She was relieved that things were going to plan. She had completed arrangements at her end and it sounded as though there would be quite a reception when I arrived the next day. There were no arrangements for the media to be there, for which I was thankful, although apparently Radio Shropshire were planning to telephone me at eight o'clock on the following morning, and the Shropshire Talking Newspaper for the Blind wanted to interview me in Shrewsbury. I didn't mind this because the volunteers who run this do a wonderful job and anyway I would be talking to many people that I know and who, perhaps, may one day benefit from my efforts.

I was more than ready for my bed when I retired at half past ten but I was determined that tomorrow's route should be clear in my mind. This study was a little different from my usual habit, since I had originally planned to walk along the B5476 from Whitchurch through Wem to Shrewsbury, but now I would have to stay on the A49 in order to meet up with Edna and the reception committee. It is no further that way, but it is a much busier road. There were no complications and soon I was able to sleep.

Day Twenty

It didn't seem long before David woke me. He gave me a cup of tea and said that breakfast would be ready in a quarter of an hour. It was then half past six. I got up immediately and was washed and dressed and had even packed some of my things before going down to breakfast. I was so keen to get started that I felt it must be obvious to everyone but I made an effort to keep calm and quiet. Wilf followed me down and we were soon tucking into our eggs, bacon, sausage, beans and tomato all expertly prepared by David, who looked as if he enjoyed doing it. We appreciated how much both David and Maira had put themselves out for us. I realised that they had not returned home from the function they had attended until after midnight, and nevertheless were up and about by six o'clock.

I think that Wilf was anxious to be on the way as well, though he never showed it. He is a person who doesn't appear to hurry or get flustered but then you suddenly realise that everything is in order and has been done, usually much more quickly and effectively than I could have done it, for all my dashing around. That was how it was this morning. I was still wondering what to do next when Wilf came into the room to say that he had packed the car and checked the bedrooms to make sure that nothing was left behind. We were supplied with coffee and sandwiches, enough to last to Land's End, never mind Shrewsbury. Then, with the log signed and the good wishes of our hosts ringing in our ears, we were off again.

It was the nineteenth of April. I reckoned that after today's walk there should be only three hundred miles to go, and that two thirds of the total distance would be behind me. I had had luck on my side until now, would it last? It would have to if I was to complete the walk by the end of the month!

The drive to the start point at Spurstow was uneventful. The volume of traffic however caused us to take much longer to get there than the same route had taken on the previous evening. It was after half past eight when I started walking. It had been raining during the night but it was dry now and the sky was brightening. The cool breeze was northerly and helpful and it seemed as if even the elements were now on my side.

This stretch of the A49 is reasonably straight with no real hills of the sort that I had met further north and with the help of the breeze I was going faster than at any other time on the walk when, near Bickley Moss, I caught my foot in something which went down with a terrific crash. When I went back to investigate I found that I had stumbled into a sign warning of road works. I reassembled it and walked warily on until the roadworks were behind me. Such things are hazards that are not marked on any map and cannot be prepared for. If it is simply a matter of painting white lines, or hedge cutting it is not much of a problem but major tasks such as drain laying or road widening may mean walking for half a mile along a narrow single carriageway with traffic coming first one way and then the other.

I passed through Whitchurch easily enough and then I had to make sure that I stayed on the A49. Although I knew I must keep on that road and I had studied the route, I still had to fight the temptation to go along the B5476 as I had originally planned.

We stopped for lunch between Prees and Prees Green. This was fifteen miles into the day's programme and it was only fourteen miles from Bayston Hill which is south of Shrewsbury and the target I had in mind. It was half past twelve so there was plenty of time, even allowing for a an hour's delay at the reception point I should be able to finish walking by six o'clock. All this we discussed as we sat trying to eat our way through the enormous repast that Maira had packed for us. We both had healthy appetites and I was eating and drinking far more than I normally did but even so it was often the case on this journey that the food put before me and provided was more than I could manage.

I suggested to Wilf that he telephone Edna and tell her that we hoped to be at the meeting point shortly after four o'clock. He said that he would also let his wife, Margaret, know that he expected be home at about six. Edna was pleased he had telephoned as she could now tell the rest of the reception committee. In fact I think she told a few others as well.

The next eight miles were behind me when I came across Wilf parked in a lay-by and talking to a lady and gentleman who he introduced as Helen and Mike Woollen. Mike was the Chairman of The Shrewsbury Branch of the Lions Association who were making a generous donation to the Fight for Sight and wanted me to accept a cheque. I was very grateful but suggested that it might be better if he presented the cheque when we reached the meeting point where it could be done formally and photographs taken. Mike was happy to do this, and asked if I would mind if he walked with me. He had already been to the meeting place and met Edna and had come out to intercept me and to accompany me the rest of the way. Mike is an experienced walker, but the conditions of walking along busy A roads was new to him.

Wilf and Helen drove off in their cars and Mike and I walked the two or three miles to the pub car park where Edna and about a dozen or so people were waiting for us. Mike had no trouble keeping up with me but the proximity of the traffic bothered him. I am sure he would have been happier in a car on this road than walking along it.

I was pleased to see so many friends. So much had happened since I had last seen any of them, yet it was less than three weeks since I had set off. Mike presented a cheque, and another was presented by Dr. Gemmell on behalf of the Shropshire Voluntary Association for the Blind. I thanked them both, and some photographs were taken. I then introduced Wilf to Eric Richards who was to be my minder when I set off again, which would be at seven o'clock on Monday morning. Then it was time to say good-bye to Wilf, and give him my heartfelt thanks for all his thoughtful support. He was by now understandably anxious to get home. The plan was that Wilf should drive to his home in Sutton Coldfield, taking Eric as a passenger, and then Eric would return in the car to his home in Shrewsbury, where he would keep it until Monday, when he would come to pick me up.

I said good-bye to Mike and his wife Helen, and then to Eric's wife, also Helen and then those of us who remained agreed to go to a cafe since we had got cold standing around. We had a relaxing drink and a chat, and then I wanted to set off to finish my day's schedule. Edna could not understand why I wanted to walk any more that day, nevertheless she agreed to meet me in an hour's time south of Shrewsbury on the A49 at Bayston Hill.

Shrewsbury is one of the easiest places of any size I know for walking around because there is a good, wide and even path for cyclists and pedestrians which is separate from the road. In fact I reached Bayston Hill in less than an hour but Edna was there waiting to drive me the fifteen miles to our cottage, and a longed for relaxing evening in my own home and familiar surroundings. Edna was surprised that I did not have a mountain of dirty washing and I explained that the good friends I had found along the route had done it all for me. She only needed to wash the clothes I was wearing.

Things seemed very normal. I had a bath while Edna prepared an evening meal. If we had thought we would be left in peace to eat it , we were soon disillusioned. The telephone started to ring and no sooner had we finished one call than it began again. Edna seemed to be quite used to this happening, and had arranged the room so that the telephone was on the table and in easy reach. The table had been moved so that it was against the wide windowsill, where the piles of maps, timetables and information about collecting and all correspondence needing replies were arranged in neat order.

Eventually we managed to finish the meal, and I volunteered to wash up, since it is one of the few ways that I can make myself useful in the kitchen. Slowly we were able to catch up on each other's news and make arrangements for the following day. The programme evolved; first there was the telephone call from Radio Shropshire at eight a.m., then I was to meet a group of friends in Bayston Hill and continue into Shrewsbury to do some collecting. After that at about half past eleven, I would return to Bayston Hill where I had stopped walking and cover the distance from there to my home. I intended to leave the A49 to take the Old Shrewsbury Road through All Stretton into Church Stretton where we would spend an hour or so collecting. I would then continue on home while Edna drove to Craven Arms and Harry Tuffin's Supermarket where three friends intended to do some collecting on my behalf. Finally we would meet up at home for a quiet evening, or so I hoped.

During the early evening the telephone continued to ring. One of the calls was from a granddaughter to say that she was coming over to visit me, along with her parents and two younger brothers. At this point I abandoned any lingering thoughts of a quiet peaceful time.

In order to keep up my schedule and leave open the possibility of completing the walk in April, I planned to walk fifteen miles on the following day, from Bayston Hill to home, and then on Sunday to walk another fifteen miles. This would be the equivalent of one day's walk in two days and the minimum needed, leaving me to average a little over thirty miles a day for the remaining nine days, a tall order. These plans I kept to myself, just saying that I wanted to walk some way on Sunday. Therefore, when Edna spoke on the telephone to the Secretary of the Bishop's Castle Rambling Group, who was asking if the group could walk a little way with me on Sunday, she agreed and suggested that they came to the cottage at half past nine. I knew that my idea of an early start and a quick march down the A49 would not now be possible and that my target of fifteen miles might be a little optimistic. However, the group had been very supportive, and one of its members was Harry Field, whose invaluable help had seen me through the first and in many ways most difficult stage, so I was not going to argue with the arrangement.

It was after eleven o'clock when we had our final telephone call of the day. It was from our daughter who had tried many times to get through and had thought that we had taken the phone off the hook to have a peaceful evening. I was able to tell her how well things were going. It had been a long and satisfying day, but tiring, and for the first time in many days I was able to go to sleep in my own bed, with no route to study. I think I was asleep before my head hit the pillow.

Day Twenty One

I woke and pressed the button on talking alarm clock and the synthesised voice told me it was six fifteen a.m. I lay there while the tea maker made the tea, a luxury that I hadn't enjoyed for some time. I thought that of all the different beds I had slept in none were as comfortable as my own. However, I couldn't lie about for long as I had a busy day ahead of me. By eight o'clock we had had breakfast, and dressed in warm clothes for the cold business of standing out in the open collecting donations. John King of Radio Shropshire called on cue at eight and after a few minutes introductory chat he asked me about the walk and its purpose. These were questions which had been put to me a number of times and I was able to explain in a few words what it was all about. I was also able to mention that we would be doing some collecting in the town that morning, I had learned from my experience in Inverness the value of Radio publicity. John King then asked me to let him know when the walk was complete, wished me success, and it was over.

Determined to help as much as they could, a couple of our oldest and closest friends arrived from Birmingham. Joan and Ron Webster had shared with us many experiences including several years of camping holidays when the children were young, the telling of which would fill a book in themselves. I remember one incident when Ron and I between us accidentally started a minor bush fire while trying to light a primus stove. The Fire Brigade arrived and wanted to know how the blaze started. We tried to look innocent and puzzled, when Ron's son proudly announced

"My dad did it !", and my son, not to be outdone, declared
"And my dad helped!"

The four of us drove cheerfully off into Shrewsbury, stopping on the way at Bayston Hill to tell our other helpers where we would be. The day was cool, and cloudy but not too unpleasant for the job we were doing. The people of Shrewsbury were generous. Many had heard the radio interview and some even came out in order to look for me. One of the reporters from the Talking Newspaper for the Blind came and spoke to me, recording what was said on a little hand held machine and I was able to hear the result when I played my tape of the next edition of the newspaper. Among the people who contributed to the cause was a man who asked incredulously if I had really walked from John O'Groats, and when I said yes, shook his head and said that if ever it occurred to him to do something like that, he would go and have a long lie down until the feeling passed.

We stopped collecting as planned at half past eleven. Carol Ray, our helper from Bayston Hill took me back to my starting point while Edna, Ron and Joan carried the tins and other collecting gear back to the car and no doubt found somewhere to have a hard earned cup of tea. I began to walk but I hadn't been going for long when a car slowed down beside me and a voice shouted before the car moved out of range. This car was in the next lay-by I came to, the driver was a colleague of mine from my working days who happened to be in the area and was intending to call on us to see how I was getting on. It was a coincidence that he and I were on the same stretch of road at the same time. There was no coincidence however involved in the appearance of the next car that slowed down as it passed with a great deal of noise and shouting. Waiting for me in the lay-by was my son and his wife and their three excited children. I told them that I had arranged to meet Edna at a pub in Dorrington which was three miles further on, where we hoped to get some lunch. They thought it would be a good idea to drive on and meet up with me there, so after a brief interlude, I was able to get on my way again.

By the time I reached Dorrington there was a drink and a ploughman's lunch waiting for me. The drink was fruit juice, as I hardly ever drink anything alcoholic because it seems to affect my ability to see and I am anxious to do nothing to interfere with the spot of vision I still have. However, I enjoy the atmosphere of a village pub and here both the food and the company were good.

There was still another nine or ten miles to walk and it was taking me a long time. It was determination rather than enthusiasm that motivated me when I set off after lunch, but after about half a mile my rhythm returned and I was moving well when my son caught up with me. He had been running then he fell into step behind me until we reached Leebotwood and turned off the A49 towards All Stretton. Here there was another delay while the photographer from the Shropshire Star persuaded me to pose by a road sign for a photograph but at last we were on the way to Church Stretton. Before we reached the village we met a group of friends two of whom gave me cheques to put in the fund. my son's wife also met up with us to tell us that Edna had gone into Craven Arms to see how the collection had gone there, and also that the Life Boat Charity was having a flag day in Church Stretton. I had no intention of interfering with their fund-raising efforts and was quite pleased that I had a valid excuse for not trying to collect there. I still had three miles to walk to reach my home and the twelve or thirteen miles I had covered so far had taken four and a half hours because of all the interruptions.

The last three miles however passed quickly. My son, Frank, continued to walk with me, and we were able to catch up on the sports news of the last three weeks so that, by the time we arrived, I was up-to-date. Edna arrived from Craven Arms at almost the same time and then immediately started to organise a meal for nine people. Christine, Frank's wife was her able assistant while Joan, as supervisor, watched the three grandchildren count the money that had been collected during the day. The children counted the money and put it meticulously into piles, each pile having a slip of paper recording the amount. We accepted their reckoning while they were there, although we checked it afterwards and found that it was exactly right. There was £236.42p from Shrewsbury and £71.15p from Craven Arms plus £50 in cheques and the children were aged five, seven and eight, so I think they did extremely well. I haven't included the age of the supervisor, Joan, but she is a little older!

While all this was going on Frank and I kept out of the way, neither of us being much of an asset in the kitchen. Fortunately as it was Saturday we could catch up with the football and rugby results. Ron who had also been shunted out of the way sat with the newspaper on his lap and his eyes shut, doing a convincing impression of a man catching up on a bit of sleep. The

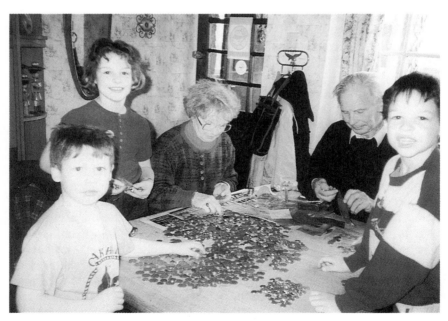

Family checking the cash collected in Shrewsbury

108

meal was a happy affair even though there was some disagreement as to whether Naomi, Richard or five year old Michael was the best money counter. They appealed to Joan for arbitration, and with a skill beyond my understanding, she managed to persuade them that they all were the best but they were not to boast about it. Soon after we had finished eating Frank and Chris decided that it was time for them to go home so they bundled the children into the car and off they went, leaving the four oldies feeling as though a hurricane had just passed. A delightful storm which nevertheless made us more than grateful for the peace it left behind.

The evening which passed all too quickly was one of those quiet pleasant times that come when in the company of true friends with common interests and a similar sense of humour. There were only a couple of telephone calls, one to say that two of my sisters and their husbands would call to see us the following afternoon to discuss their part as my minders for the last stage of the walk. This was good news for me for I find it much easier to make arrangements face to face than by telephone. I did spend a little time looking at my route before going to sleep that night but it was more for the purpose of finding a realistic target for the day than to examine the route, with which I was already familiar.

Day Twenty Two

All four of us were up bright and early on that Sunday morning. We had a good cooked breakfast and were already booted and looking forward to a pleasant walk when eight of our friends from the Bishop's Castle Rambling Group arrived promptly at half past nine. The walk I had planned was a pleasant meander through the lanes in the general direction of Craven Arms. The Shropshire countryside is, to me, wonderful at any time of year and in April and May it is at its best.

As we walked the birds were singing their hearts out, I'm sure they sing all the louder and sweeter for me as if they know I can't see them. Because I know where to look, I found primroses and daffodils, now perhaps a little past their best, campions, ragworts celandine, white dead nettle, cowslips, bluebells and a host of spring flowers. The flowers were sometimes growing singly and sometimes grouped together and on occasion they covered the ground in a carpet of colour. Snowdrops, a particular favourite, were finished, but you can't have everything!

The oilseed rape was coming into flower, soon there would be great patches of bright yellow dominating the landscape. I noticed that crops were more advanced here than they had been further north, and this one particularly. I suppose it is because there are so many of these yellow fields that they seem unnatural to me, like scars on a pretty face.

The first mile or so took us down a narrow lane much of which is sunken with steep banks rising either side to the fields. These banks revealing the roots of trees that cling on to life precariously, defying nature and the law of gravity. Some of these trees are big and old with tangled, knotted roots. They have probably been here since this same narrow lane was the main route into Wales. I have since seen one of these great trees cut down and turned into firewood with a chainsaw. A sad sight, a tree fifty foot high and four foot in diameter brought crashing down into the lane before being cut up, the torn out roots leaving a crater at the roadside big enough to drive a car into.

Back to the morning's walk. We did not get along very fast. Twice I stopped to speak to farmers that I knew, at this time keeping a careful watch over their lamb ewes. There were some lambs already but generally the local hill farmers like to have the grass growing before their Kerrys and Cluns produce their offspring. They obviously have some old wisdom that tells them such things, I know that it seems to me that the grass in my garden never actually stops growing!

The pattern of life in this area is one that always allows a few minutes chat no matter how pressing or urgent the business in hand. This is one of the pleasures of living here and one that has not changed for many years and I hope that I don't see a change in my lifetime. We had thought nothing of leaving the house unlocked with a note on the table for our expected visitors, something that would be possible in few neighbourhoods in this day and age. We passed a box full of free range eggs with a notice and a tin to pay for any eggs taken. Such things are a constant pleasure to someone like me who spent so much of my time in a city where life is a race against the clock and where a burglar alarm is almost a standard fitting for the house.

The walking party came to a halt again when someone noticed a spotted woodpecker. It was pointed out to us all, and the others watched him as he ignored the intruders and got on with his wood pecking. I tried hard but was unable to make him out.

The next three miles of the walk took us through lanes along the top of a high ridge. To the east there was the ridge of Wenlock Edge leading south towards the Clee Hills and to the west were the mountains of Wales. The weather was cool and clear with slats of sunshine filtering through a light but cloud covered sky. It was a good day for walking and a good walk for talking.

We reached Wistanstow at half past eleven. This was where I planned to continue alone. I left the others admiring the village hall, a large and elegant black and white building that might be the envy of any town yet in this case served a village of two or three hundred inhabitants. I had marked the rest of the walk on a pathfinder map, so that they could return across the fields, making it a circular walk of about ten miles. I then carried on towards Craven Arms before turning off along the old Watling Street. After a while this narrows to a path, cut by the Shrewsbury to South Wales railway line. Over the fence, a careful listen for trains, a quick dash then over the fence on the other side. I was then back on the path that was once one of the main roads of Roman Britain.

I passed a small encampment of travellers or gypsies and noticed piles of scrap, or burnt patches where they had lit fires. I heard the furious barking of dogs and this helped to add a mile an hour to my speed even though, thank goodness! the dogs were chained up.

Two hundred yards further and I reached the junction with the next lane, where the Watling street becomes a highway for half a mile, before transforming once again into a narrow lane. It is three miles to the B4385 and on the map it looks absolutely straight but I had walked this way before and I knew that it twisted and turned.

Three quarters of an hour later I was on the B4385 heading towards

Leintwardine and it was two o'clock. I had asked Ron to pick me up at two, but he was a little late as it had taken the main party longer to get back than they had thought. This was good, for it enabled me to reach Leintwardine which was the objective I had had in mind.

We returned to the cottage which was noisy and cheerfully crowded since by this time my sisters Marjorie and Dorothy with Maurice and Douglas their husbands had arrived. I suggested that we sit down together and plan our strategy for the point when they would join me on the walk. I was told however that they had already sorted everything out with Edna, and all I had to do was to tell them when and where to meet me. At first I was a bit upset, feeling that things had been taken out of my control but on reflection I realised that my reaction was unfair since they were trying to reduce the pressure on me as far as they could with the areas that didn't involve the actual walking.

I still felt fresh and physically relaxed but in fact I had found the weekend hard work having to be in the right place at the right time, being interviewed, meeting and trying to recognise people, and also I found fund-raising quite tiring. I had said nothing about this but I think Edna had noticed that I was becoming exhausted by the constant mental pressure and aided and abetted by my brother-in-law, was trying to do everything she could to help.

The Rover Company had telephoned to find out where their car would be on the following Friday morning, when they expected to collect it. They had been given Eric's address. This meant that he would have to leave me on Thursday to get home in time. With this in mind we arranged that I would tell Edna when I telephoned on Wednesday where we would be at three o'clock on Thursday afternoon. They would then arrange to meet us there and transfer my belongings to their car so that Eric would be free to return home.

Edna was also going to join us at that point, and she would drive down with Maurice who had broken an ankle while sledging with his grandchildren in the snow of the winter, and therefore could not drive. His job was to be the navigator.

From that point in the walk, Maurice and Douglas would have the task of escorting me, and we would return after each day's walking to the ladies, wherever they happened to be. This plan seemed straightforward enough but experience had taught me that things seldom work out exactly as planned. The ladies were looking forward to having some time to do their own thing in Cornwall and Devon, while we were getting on with covering the miles.

By nine o'clock all the visitors had gone leaving Edna and me alone at last to enjoy a peaceful evening. In fact it was quite a hectic two or three hours since there were still frequent phone calls and we had to make preparations for the next part of the journey. Food and clean clothes were put ready to be packed into the car with a minimum of trouble. I studied and learned the next day's route. It had been a wearing weekend and I mentioned that when this was all over we deserved a holiday. Edna was pleased about that, for she had been thinking the same thing and had chosen a holiday in Austria, twelve days of hill and mountain walking in the Alps. It might not sound a very restful holiday but it was just the sort of thing I liked and I knew it would be refreshing and relaxing.

Day Twenty Three

Monday the twenty second of April saw us up and dressed by six o'clock. Edna ,despite going on a bit about getting up 'in the middle of the night' cooked breakfast for me. While for me it is natural to get up and get moving as soon as my eyes are open in the morning, for Edna it is a more gradual process. However we were ready and waiting for Eric when he arrived a minute or two before seven and we had packed and were on our way by ten minutes past. It was a beautiful spring morning, cool, still and bright with the sun rising into a cloudless sky. We stopped the car at the place where Ron had caught up with me the day before and I started walking from there. It was twenty minutes to eight. It was a relief to be on my way again.

Once through Leintwardine I turned off the B4385 on to the A4110 which, although it is an A road, is not a busy one since most of the traffic stays on the A49 which runs in the same direction a few miles to the east. Both roads lead to Hereford and the distance is about the same so the opportunity of a quieter walk was not one to be missed. I hadn't been walking for long when I almost trod on something which at first glance looked like a sleeping animal. It was a badger curled up at the roadside and looking undamaged but it was a sleep that it would not wake from. It was impossible to tell whether it had died naturally or whether it had been hit by a vehicle like so many of the other creatures that I tried to step over on this and every other day.

I had debated with myself whether to stay on the Watling Street from Leintwardine to Wigmore as it is a pleasant grassy track but I decided that I couldn't spare the extra time it would take and this road was a good one for walking. It was quiet, well-surfaced and had hedges to either side with plenty of birds singing. I even heard a cuckoo, the first of the year for me.

In the next ten miles as I passed out of Shropshire and into Herefordshire I went through a number of attractive, unspoilt little villages, Adforton, Wigmore, Yatton, Aymstrey and Mortimores Cross each with their church and pub. The houses were mainly timber framed or stone, some were thatched but not many. The sun was shining and I felt privileged to be in such a place on such a wonderful morning. After two and a half hours I had a brief stop and time to discuss progress with Eric. He had been keeping with me so far and was surprised that I had covered ten miles so far. He was now satisfied that I was alright, and felt able to drive on about four miles at a time and meet up with me every hour. This was the system Wilf had used and it worked well. I was pleased that Eric agreed since I feel it is a great strain on the driver to do any more.

I crossed the A44 at Shirl Heath then the A4112 at Stretford Court continuing towards Hereford on what was now the A4110. This was the same route that the Romans had taken through this attractive and historically interesting part of England. At one o'clock we stopped for lunch at a place called Holmer about a mile or so north of Hereford, remarkable only in that it is where another Roman road intersects going from east to west.

After lunch Eric drove off intending to park on the south side of the town and walk back to meet me while I walked into the town. Before Eric reached me However, I came to a very busy ring road which I needed to cross. As I stood at the kerb side trying to make out if there was a crossing nearby a very deep voice said in my ear;

"Are you in trouble man? Do you want to cross the road?"

I said that I did and he put a huge hand on my shoulder and we stepped onto the road. The traffic must have stopped, and my heart almost did! We reached the other side of the road and with a friendly pat my guide left me. I turned in time to see an enormous coloured man, dreadlocks flapping about his head walking straight across the road ignoring the traffic that dodged about him. I never saw his face.

Eric found me and we walked across the bridge over the river Wye and out of the town to where he had left the car. I didn't say anything about the road crossing incident, it didn't seem real somehow. It had only lasted a few seconds and when I tried to think about it afterwards I couldn't remember being aware of the traffic going around us as it surely must have done. I continued on for another three miles until I met up with Eric again. He was waiting at Kingsthorne to show me where the A466 road that I wanted forked right towards Monmouth, the A49 continuing towards Ross-on Wye. Kingsthorne had been my target for the day but it was only half past three and any further miles covered today would be a bonus so I revised my plans. My new objective was to be St. Weonards which was six miles further south and I suggested to Eric that he went on and tried to find somewhere for us to stay.

When I reached St. Weonards Eric was waiting for me, concerned because he had not been able to find anywhere that could accommodate us. The people at the Old Vicarage which normally offered B&B were unable to help as the lady of the house was ill. Eric had driven around and searched the local villages but he had drawn a blank. This was strange as we were on the edge of the beautiful Forest of Dean an area that attracts many tourists. We decided that the sensible thing to do was to go on to Monmouth where we would be sure to find a place to rest our weary heads but it was not that easy.

We drove round for a while before we found a small hotel, it was very expensive compared to some of the places I had stayed, nevertheless we would have booked in had our reception been less offhand. There were alterations being done in the corridors and foyer and carpets and materials were in piles on the floor. This together with a frosty reception made Eric bridle and I agreed that we weren't that desperate yet. As we left, Eric noticed a board in the window of a house opposite that said B&B Vacancies.

A pleasant young woman showed us clean and comfortable rooms, not very big but we agreed that they would suit us very well. We were soon installed, showered and changed and ready to go in search of something to eat. First we needed to telephone and report our progress. The first kiosk we tried would not accept coins, the next one threw them out again and I was beginning to think that Monmouth was not my favourite town, when we found a third phone box where the phone was working properly. There was not much news which was not surprising since we had only left home that morning. It was good to hear that money had been arriving by post from people who had heard the radio interview. The organisers of The Fight for Sight still wanted me to have a car phone and wanted to know where they could meet me. I said that I would be at Tintern Abbey some time on the following afternoon.

Food was our next priority. This seemed almost as difficult as finding a telephone that worked. The first place that we looked in didn't appeal to us, the second one we came to didn't cook on Mondays but at last we managed to find a fish and chip restaurant that served us with good portions in an efficient and pleasant manner. We then called in to one of the local hostelries for a quiet drink before returning to the house. It was a dark interior and not very warm so we didn't stay long. My eyes were bothering me a little, I think the messing about we had done in Monmouth after a long day walking into the sun had been too much for them. I kept this to myself, there was no point in bothering Eric who had calmly sorted out each problem as it arose and made things easy for me. I knew from experience that tomorrow would bring some problem with my eyes. How bad it would be I had no way of knowing. At worst, I would be sick, unable to focus on anything and unable to think clearly and certainly unable to walk. The best I could hope for was the nuisance of a continual ache which nevertheless would permit me to keep moving.

Back at the boarding house I tried, not very successfully, to study my map. I suggested to Eric that I would try to get up early and set off from

Monmouth towards Chepstow in order to give myself a chance to get going in the best possible conditions. He would then bring be back to Monmouth for breakfast and afterwards take me back to St. Weonards to do the six or seven miles I would have missed out. It was only ten o'clock but I excused myself, took a couple of paracetamol and went to bed, leaving Eric watching the television.

Day Twenty Four

I woke up at five o'clock with my eyes aching. I lay for a while wondering whether to try and go on. With an effort I got up and dressed and had a cup of tea from the flask I had prepared the night before. I went out of the house, it was still dark and I couldn't see a thing. Unable to go back in because I had shut the door behind me and unwilling to stand around waiting for daylight I set out to find my way out of the town. In our quest for a working telephone we had walked through a large public car park behind the house where we were staying and Eric has pointed out a path which led from it to the road which I wanted. I cautiously made my way round the house and across the car park, using the traffic noise and lights from busy A40 which I knew I had to cross, as a guide. It seemed an extremely busy road, even at that hour. Eventually, just as the first streaks of daylight appeared I reached the traffic lights at the junction of the A40 and the A466. This was the road I wanted so after what seemed like an age of waiting the traffic lights turned to green I crossed the A40 and set off along the A466.

The road I was on crossed the River Wye and then followed its meandering for the next fifteen miles along what is arguably the most beautiful valley road in the country. As I walked on that morning the beauty of my surroundings was far from my mind. I tried to concentrate on where the road edge was but it was difficult as my eyes were aching, not unbearably, but enough to make me feel miserable and sorry for myself. My legs felt heavy as I ambled along at a relatively slow pace, content under the circumstances to be moving at all. It was while in this stupor that I had a shock. Something seemed to burst out of the hedge and attack me. I could hear the beating of wings and feel the air in my face as I instinctively crossed my arms protectively in front of it. The noise subsided and I opened my eyes. I think there was a large white bird flying away. On reflection it was probably a barn owl that I had disturbed in that half light, maybe I had nearly trodden on it. One thing for certain is that I was the more scared of the two of us. This incident brought me back to reality for a while but didn't improve my well-being. If it had happened the day before I might have enjoyed it but today everything was trouble and I was concerned that I may not reach Tintern and in fact that it might be necessary to give up for the day and stay in Monmouth. This thought depressed me but I was only too aware that my legs were leaden and once or twice I stopped walking and debated whether to sit down for a while and rest. I resisted the temptation and plodded on feeling thoroughly disheartened. I knew this area well, having spent a lot of time camping and walking in the Forest of Dean and I had anticipated really enjoying this part of the journey with the River Wye on one side of me and Offa's Dyke on the other. Instead I was wishing that Eric would appear soon to take me back to the boarding house where it seemed I would have to stay for the rest of the day.

I reached the single carriageway bridge and walked across it and through Llandogo or it would be more accurate to say under it as the village seems to be perched on the high and steep hillside overlooking the road and the river which was now on my left. Eric caught up with me shortly after this and even in my present state I was cheered when he said that he had clocked seven miles from Monmouth. It was not yet eight o'clock. I had covered seven miles in two and a half hours. It was not good by my usual standard, but much better than I thought I was doing so I was pleased.

A ride back to Monmouth, a wash in cold water and five minutes to sit down made me feel better. My eyes still ached and it was an effort to eat but I did manage some breakfast. Not my usual plate-clearing job, but better than nothing and enough to keep me going. I waited until the children of the house had finished in the bathroom and gone off to school which gave me another chance of a short rest and by the time we eventually set off with the log signed and the flask filled, there was more life in my legs and I felt that perhaps I would be able to keep going. Eric had realised that my eyes were troubling me but I did not tell him how close I had been to giving up for the day.

The six or so miles from St. Weonards to the bridge out of Monmouth on the A466 where I had started that morning took me nearly two hours to walk. With my mouth clamped tightly shut I forced one leg in front of the other, determined now that I would get to Tintern that day. As Monmouth came into sight I began to feel some rhythm in my step and the pain in my right eye had definitely eased. Eric had a drink ready for me when I reached the car. He had not been at all bothered by the length of time it had taken me to walk that last section, and I was glad that I was not still with Harry or Wilf, who would have expected me at least half an hour earlier. From my previous stopping point I planned to walk the remaining two miles to Tintern while he drove on to see if the people from the Fight for Sight had arrived at the meeting place.

When I was half a mile from Tintern a young woman approached me and introduced herself as Ann. I had spoken to her several times by telephone as she worked for the Fight for Sight Charity. We walked into Tintern together and she told me that she had been fund-raising at an Optical Seminar and Fair at the N.E.C. in Birmingham and had thought she would take the opportunity to meet up with me to take a few photographs and to offer me a car phone on loan. I didn't mind the photographs but I didn't want the car phone which I was told was expensive to use and had to be well looked after. We reached the place where the cars were parked and I met two other young women who were with Ann. We spent about ten minutes talking and taking photographs and had to convince them that a car phone would be more of a liability than an asset. They wished me luck, said good-bye and drove off. Maybe it was because I was still not feeling very good, but I couldn't help wondering about the cost of sending three young women in an expensive high performance hired car a hundred miles out of their way to lend me a car phone that I did not want! And I couldn't help thinking of the effort required to raise such an amount!

Eric and I had lunch and wandered down to the Abbey to have a look at what is left of the still imposing building, for once I was not filled with urgency to be on my way. We had both been here before, so after a brief tour round I set off again. The break had done me good, my left eye still ached but compared to what I had put up with that morning it was a minor problem.

The valley road continues for two miles south of Tintern until, near St. Arvans the River Wye turns east to join the River Severn. We were

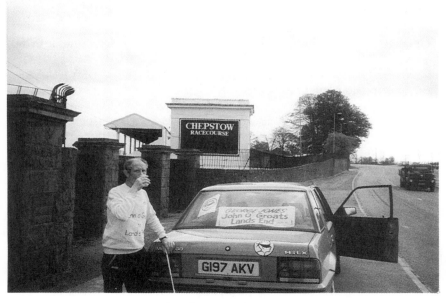

Another watering stop

120

approaching the Severn Bridge and needed to work out a plan for crossing it and meeting on the other side. Eric waited for me at the entrance to Chepstow Racetrack, a wide and convenient place to park. He said that there was a Services Area on the Bristol side of the bridge where he would meet me.

It was fortunate for me that Eric had foreseen difficulties for me on the approach to the bridge and that he had waited for me there. He was able to direct me along a rather complicated route to the footbridge which involved walking along a narrow field path before crossing under the M4 to the walkway which is on the south side of the bridge. There was no-one about to ask so it would have taken me a long time to sort it out without help. This kind of thoughtfulness is typical of Eric who was organised and considerate and seemed to have a knack of anticipating my problems, and knowing when I needed help and when I could manage alone. The fact that he has a daughter, now married and with a family of her own, who is registered blind may account for his sensitivity.

It was a full half hour before I saw Eric again. He was waiting at the end of the walkway and led me to the Service Area where the car was parked. Over a cup of coffee we discussed the next move. I had enjoyed the walk over the bridge, the weather was fine but breezy as I suspect it usually is, being open to the estuary. The crossing seemed to be in two sections. I had been going for some distance and thought I was across when I reached a steel structure when I saw below me the narrow channel of water that is all that is left of this great river when the tide is out. Then I realised that I was only half way across.

While we sat drinking our coffee Eric mentioned that I looked better. Sometime during that crossing my eye had stopped aching and I hadn't noticed. Suddenly I felt fit and started talking about getting to Bristol that day, but Eric, knowing me better than I did myself at that moment said that he thought I had struggled through a long hard day and that after he had seen me away from the bridge and onto the right road he should go and find us somewhere to stop for the night. He was right of course and after leading me back under the M4 and onto the A403 he returned to the car, passing me a few moments later on his way to finding us a lodging for the night.

Two miles down the A403 and just before Severn Beaches I turned inland on a road signposted to Easter Compton and Bristol. Eric met me then and he was walking, having left the car at the place he had found, half a mile away at Pilning. This was far enough for me. In a broken, messy day of travelling I had covered twenty five miles, twice as far as I had thought possible a few hours earlier and I was still on schedule.

As we walked the last half mile Eric told me that it wasn't much of a place he had found but it was clean and there was a pub down the road where we could get a meal. Imagine my surprise therefore when we turned down a long drive through a pretty and well-tended garden and went into a large and very attractive house. We were welcomed by a smiling lady who told us to make ourselves comfortable while she made us a cup of tea or coffee.

I looked at Eric who smiled and winked, enjoying my amazement at our palatial surroundings and said;

"Wait until you see the bedrooms!"

They were really worth waiting to see, we each had a large, tastefully decorated room with en-suite bathroom and even the cups and saucers provided with the facilities for making drinks in the rooms were of bone china. It was real luxury.

The days journey had finished by five o'clock, and the prospect of a long leisurely evening was appealing to both of us. While I was enjoying a long soak in the bath I noticed that the toenails of the little toes on each of my feet had turned black! They were not sore or painful but they were definitely black. There was no reason for this that I could think of, I kept my nails clipped and short and had felt no foot discomfort during the day.

There was ample time to study my next day's route as I sat in a comfortable chair , coffee to hand enjoying the peace. It occurred to me that I felt hungry and I pressed the button on my talking clock and the voice told me that it was six twenty p.m. I went off in search of a telephone to make my calls before finding somewhere to eat. I asked Mrs. Truscott, at whose house we were staying to direct us to a public telephone but she insisted that we use her private telephone. This instrument sat on the hall table and was a portable telephone which I had no idea how to use. After several minutes of pressing and switching to no effect, I found someone nearby and asked for help. An attractive young woman dialled my home number for me and read out to me the telephone number of the house so that I could relay it to Edna and she could call me back. I told Edna where we were and was about to tell her that I had managed to meet up with the ladies from Fight for Sight when she told me that they had telephoned her to say that I was doing fine. I bet they used the car phone to make the call!

Edna was still very busy and was looking forward to joining me as it would be a short holiday for her, a rest after the hurly-burly of the last week or three. She was also trying to keep abreast of the work in the garden so that she could leave it looking tidy when she left on Thursday.

There was about half an hour to spare before the time we had planned to go out for an evening meal and we spent it talking with the family. I learned that Mrs. Truscott's eldest daughter had a detached lens rendering her virtually blind in one eye and while the sight of the other eye was good, the lens connection was tenuous. This was the young woman who had been so helpful to me by explaining the complications of the portable telephone. Among the guest at the house was a woman from New Zealand who had come to Europe on a sight-seeing tour. She said it would be her last chance to travel in freedom as she was getting married on her return home. We were still chatting to her when the time came for us to go out for our meal. She was interesting company and we were pleased when she agreed to join us.

It was a clear, cool evening and we walked briskly to the local inn. Once there was no more hurry and rush. A cheery log fire burned in the grate and we sat, lit by its flickering, enjoying a relaxing drink and deciding what we would eat. A spell in the equally comfortable dining room, and suitably replenished we returned to the cosy lounge which by that time had filled up a little, and we sat with the hum of relaxed conversation in the background while we finished a drink before strolling back to the house.

Before I went to bed, we had coffee and biscuits in the lounge and spoke with a couple of business men who said they always stayed with Mrs. Truscott when they were in the area and who could blame them. It really was the most comfortable and welcoming place. I was tired however and did not linger for long. I felt pleased that I had the route for the following day in my mind and I went to sleep thinking how lucky it was to have had such a good end to a day which had started off so badly.

Day Twenty Five

I had told the Truscotts that I liked to walk before breakfast and at six o'clock I let myself out of the house and into the still, cool morning. I felt fit and well, a complete contrast to the way I had felt setting out the day before. The first two miles were along a quiet suburban road through Easter Compton as far as the M5 motorway. I came to a roundabout with roads off to the motorway, both north and south and I knew I had to be careful to avoid those. I safely negotiated my way past the entry to the M5 north and turned onto a wide road that I thought would lead me to the Clifton area of Bristol and to the suspension bridge which I had to cross. I had an uneasy feeling that something was wrong but I couldn't think what it might be. The picture in my mind was quite clear - at the roundabout go past the motorway entry and take the next road on the left. This was what I had done. The road was very quiet and I could hear traffic noise on my right and behind me. This told me that something was definitely wrong. The noise from behind me was the traffic on the motorway and that was as it should be, the nearest main road on my right however, should be the A4 Avonmouth road, which was at least a mile away. I was aware of this because at one stage I had contemplated going through Avonmouth after crossing the Severn Bridge and then walking to Clifton on the A4.

Fortunately soon after I realised this a man's voice wished me

"Good morning"

If he had not spoken to me I would not have noticed him. I was able to ask him if I was on the right road into Bristol. I was not. By the time I got back to the M4 roundabout I had spent more than half an hour walking around the maze of an industrial estate not marked on my map.

Once back to the roundabout I continued on until I found the next exit which was the right road. Eric passed me and parked a little way ahead, waiting for me and we went back for breakfast. It was eight o'clock and I had only walked five miles.

We ate breakfast in a room with a large patio window looking out over a pretty flower bordered lawn with two wild rabbits scampering about on it completely ignoring the large dog which lay on the patio watching them. Mrs. Truscott said that they did eat some of her plants and that it would be a waste of time growing vegetables but the rabbits were so much a part of the garden that she would not try to get rid of them. The breakfast was like everything else in that house, very good. The long evening after yesterday's early finish had contributed to the feeling that this stop was like a short holiday and both Eric and I felt better for our stay with this lovely family. We had to get on. We paid our bill and gratefully accepted a donation to our cause which was added to the two we had been given at the pub last evening when our New Zealand friend told several people what I was doing. We left the house, with log signed and supplied with coffee and sandwiches at the same time as Mrs Truscott who was taking her two younger children to school. We paused only for a short photographic session and set off to the spot where Eric had picked me up before breakfast.

After half an hour of walking I reached the Clifton Suspension Bridge. I am quite pleased that when I looked down I could not make out the water so far below me as I made my way across the Isambard Kingdom Brunel's famous bridge. At the southern side of the bridge Eric was waiting for me and we walked together until he was sure that I was on the right road, the A38 when he returned to collect the car. He soon passed me and the next time we met was five miles along the road near to Bristol Airport. By now the weather had changed, it was drizzling and there was a southerly breeze making a nuisance of itself, forcing the wetness into my face. I was reluctant to put on my waterproofs, I had got out of the habit of wearing them but it soon became obvious that they were necessary as the drizzle turned to rain.

After about an hour the rain stopped and I was thankful to discard my waterproofs. It was a little early but as we had stopped we decided to have lunch. I was now going well. I had passed through Redhill over the Congresbury Yeo River and I was a mile north of Churchill. Lower Langford was on the right and the Mendip Hills on my left. It started to rain heavily while we were eating. so much for my hopes of putting away the waterproof gear! We extended the break a little in the hope that the rain might ease off but there was no sign of it so of I went with my coat and leggings on and my hood up trying to peer through the curtain of rain in front of my eyes and realising that I had not fully appreciated my good fortune in having twelve rain-free days in April. It was an hour and a half later when I passed the turn off to Axbridge and Cheddar Gorge. A long hour and a half in which I had only covered five miles. A combination of wearing waterproofs and a lack of urgency had caused my speed to drop and though it didn't matter because we had decided to stop for the night at Highbridge which was eight miles away, it was already three o'clock and I didn't want to start getting into the bad habit of slowing down, besides, I appreciated the long evening rest after a day which finished early.

The next time I caught up with Eric was when he stopped about four miles from Highbridge near where the A38 crosses the M5 motorway at

Rook's Bridge. After a quick coffee, Eric went on to find a night's lodging. This could not have taken him very long because he met me at Edithead and walked with me for the last mile to the place where we were to stay. He had booked in at the Highbridge Hotel which was on the A38, convenient for me as it meant that I didn't have to find my way in the morning. The room I had was warm and comfortable. Unfortunately the stairs and corridors were not well enough lit for me to see. A dim light is attractive and acceptable in such a traditional inn but for me it is as bad as no light at all.

We ordered an evening meal for half past seven giving me plenty of time to have a bath, change , study the map and make telephone calls. The map study was more important even than usual as I had to find a place convenient to meet Edna and the others for the changeover of drivers and to estimate what time I would get there. It had to be somewhere that was easy to find and where three cars could park. I decided that the approach road to junction 26 of the M5 at West Boland would fit the bill and after working out the distance I thought I should be able to get there by half past two which would give Eric a chance to leave in order to get home at a reasonable time. I asked Eric to check my distance calculations and estimated times and to tell me what he thought. He agreed that the meeting place was suitable but as the distance was twenty six miles he thought I should allow more time to get there. We decided to leave it as it was however and if I was behind schedule I could always get to the meeting place by car.

Having worked that out I knew that I needed to give the actual route more attention than usual as well. Although the whole day would be along the A38 and was straightforward in that respect, the road led through Bridgewater and Taunton, both big enough to cause me problems if I didn't keep my wits about me. I was satisfied that my mental picture was clear enough before I went to find a telephone at just after six o'clock. Edna had been eagerly waiting for my call. I explained the plan twice and then repeated it more slowly a third time so that she could write it down. I then asked her to read it back to me so that there would be no error. Edna was enthusiastic about joining me, she said that, my calls excepted, she was fed up with the constant ringing of the telephone and was really looking forward to getting away from it for a few days. I knew that she would have several more calls to make that evening so I didn't spend my usual time asking questions, knowing that we could catch up on the news soon enough.

It had stopped raining and Eric and I wandered around Highbridge. It was still a damp and dismal evening and we were glad to get back to the warmth and comfort of the bar at the Highbridge Hotel. The place was empty except for the hotelier and his wife and we sat on high stools at the bar putting the world to rights for half an hour before other customers and duties called them away. Among the things we discussed was the weather and they told us that the forecast for the following day was for showers and longer periods of rain. This disturbed me a bit for the prospect of trying to keep to my timetable while battling with the hated waterproof gear was daunting. It made me all the more determined to make an early start. When I told the hotelier of my plans he just grinned and told me to make sure the door was shut behind me.

I enjoyed the meal which we ate in the bar which was neither crowded nor smoke-filled. We were sitting with a drink at about nine o'clock when Eric suggested a stroll down to see the boats on the river. Highbridge is only a mile from Burnham-on-Sea and the mouth of the River Brue which flows through Highbridge into Bridgewater Bay is apparently a popular tie-up point. Although I wasn't particularly tired I decided not to go with him mainly because of the risk of straining my eyes trying to see in the dark - the walk from Monmouth to the Severn Bridge was still fresh in my mind - but also I wanted an early night in order to have an early start. Eric had not returned by the time I went to bed at ten o'clock and I did not see him again until he came to bring me back for breakfast the next morning. Once in my room I quickly checked the route then set my alarm for half past five. I had not done this before since I normally have no trouble waking up at the time I want. I wanted to be sure of getting as far as possible before breakfast.

Day Twenty six

The next morning when I woke and pressed the button on my clock it told me that it was five twenty a.m. I put the switch over to prevent the alarm sounding and got up, wide awake and eager to be on my way. Having a room to myself meant that I could put the light on without disturbing anyone. The kettle boiled while I was getting washed and dressed and all was well. Then I heard the rain beating on the window and looked out. All I could see was a starry halo around each of the street lights and otherwise all was dark. Some of my enthusiasm evaporated, especially since I had to put on the dreaded waterproofs and it took me a while longer than usual to drink my tea. With an effort I left the well-lit room and emerged into the corridor feeling around for an elusive light switch until I gave up trying to find one. Trying to be as quiet as I could I crept along the corridor and went through a doorway to the stairs The floorboards in this old building didn't just creak, they squealed. The stairs were less of a problem than the corridor, for like many visually handicapped people I automatically counted them on the way up. The stairs led into an entrance hall with several doors leading off it. Once again I could not locate a light switch. I felt my way to each door in turn running my hands around them to find a bolt or something that would tell me that this was the door which led to the road. The harder I tried to be quiet the more noise I seemed to make. When I got back to the stairs for the second time, I decided to make my way to my room to collect my torch and slowly creaked my way back. Fortunately I had remembered how many doors there were between the top of the stairs and my room so it wasn't very long before I had collected the torch and with its help I soon reached the hall and unbolted the main door.

It was ten minutes to six on the twenty fifth of April when I stepped out into that very wet street determined to get as good a start as possible despite the weather. One consolation was that the amount of time it had taken me to get out of the Hotel meant that the sky was a few shades lighter. I could see the road edge, there was no traffic about, in fact there was nothing and no-one about and I felt as though I were the only living thing on the planet as I hurried down the main road out of that silent place. It must have been a full ten minutes before the first car went passed. I had just reached Huntspill which confirmed that I was on the right road. The absence of traffic had made me think that perhaps I had wandered onto some Trading Estate by mistake as I had the day before. As the rain eased and the light improved my spirits rose and I was moving along well. Even when I found myself in a ditch having temporarily lost the road edge where a wide field gate entrance coincided with a right hand bend in the road and I had continued on straight forward, I picked myself up and there was no damage done and no time lost. I am usually so embarrassed when that sort of thing happens that I jump straight up and carry on hoping that no-one has seen me tumble. I am accustomed to ignoring the odd scratch or bruise caused by such things and in this case all I had sustained was one wet foot.

The weather continued to improve until, at Dunball, after an hour and a half, the rain stopped and I gratefully climbed out of my leggings. At this

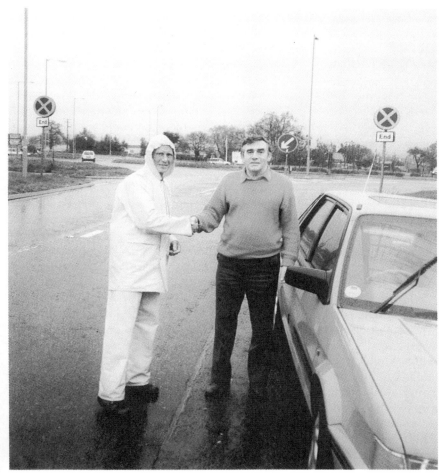

(Devon) Goodbye to Eric

place the A38 comes close to the M5 junction 23 before forking away towards Bridgewater and I stood for a minute watching, even at this hour, the endless streams of traffic and wondered what it would have been like on this road had the motorway not been built.

It was with a feeling of relief that I crossed the River Parrett some time later and turned left towards Taunton. Bridgewater was now behind me and I had managed to get through using my mental picture with no problems. The position of the river confirmed that I was still on the right road and I could get on with the next part of the walk. Once again the A38 came close to the M5 at junction 24, about a mile south of Bridgewater, and another of my reference points was behind me. The next would be North Petherton.

Before I reached North Petherton Eric passed me and pulled into a convenient gateway. It was five past eight and I was nine miles into the day's journey. Back in Highbridge I had breakfast, put on dry socks and boots and then went to see if I could find an explanation for the difficulty I had had finding the right door that morning. There seemed to be no reason, except possibly that the stairs came into the hallway at an angle which may have upset my perspective. This trivial incident bothered me and was a blow to my confidence. How could I have failed to find the door? I found myself thinking about it several times during the day and wondering if the lapse in concentration was a one-off occurrence or a signal that days of mental effort were beginning to tell. Physically I felt fine but my head was full of numbers and figures and there were times when I would have liked a break from thinking and planning. This sort of bothering was a nuisance, it did nothing for my confidence and encouraged a feeling at the back of my mind that something was going to go wrong. I was not unduly morbid or afraid but I thought that I had had more than my share of good fortune and expected something to come along to balance this.

Eric organised the packing of the car. Our hosts, Susan and Bruno Fellman, signed the log and we were on our way. When I began to walk the miserable drizzle was not much of a handicap so I did not bother to wear my leggings. According to my reckoning Highbridge was one hundred and sixty one miles from Land's End and my self-imposed schedule left five and a half days. This would be fine as long as there were no major complications or miscalculations. I had already done nine of them and the next seven, from North Petherton to Taunton were behind me by half past eleven. Eric was waiting as I approached Taunton. This was near to junction 25 of the M5. These junction numbers had become important to me as they marked my progress. Eric steered me through the town leaving me to return to the car only when he was sure that I was on the A38 going towards Wellington and more significantly towards West Buckland and junction 26.

The next time Eric caught up with me we decided to have lunch. We had time to spare as we were only three miles from the meeting point and had two hours to get there. It was on with the waterproofs again as I set off after an extended lunch break. The drizzle had turned to steady rain. I arrived at junction 26 three quarters of an hour early and I was pleased to get out of the rain and wait in the car with Eric.

At exactly half past two Edna drove up behind us. She arrived with Maurice and explained that Douglas and my two sisters Marjorie and Dorothy were unpacking and settling into the caravan they had found for us to stay in. This was at Westward Ho. Eric had already separated his gear so that we could easily transfer everything else into our car which Edna was driving. This done we said our farewells, and I expressed my very genuine thanks to Eric for the way he had looked after me. He set off then for home.

Edna and Maurice were a little taken aback when I said that I wanted to carry on walking. They had thought that as it was raining I would be glad to stop and go back to the caravan with them. As I was putting on my leggings and waterproof jacket, Edna said that she had intended to take a photograph of Eric and me at the changeover. It was then I remembered where the camera was. We had been taking photographs regularly in order to create a record of the walk and the last time I had done this I had put the camera in the passenger door pocket of Eric's car. Just then a car pulled in. Eric had spotted the camera before he reached the motorway and had come back to hand it over. The photograph was taken and I set off.

I carried on walking until five o'clock. By then I had walked through Wellington and on to Appledore. Despite the changeover and the continuous rain I reckoned that I had covered thirty four miles.

It was about forty miles by car to Westward Ho and I was quite content to sit back and relax in the back of the car as Edna drove and Maurice navigated. The trip took longer than it ought to have done as we had trouble locating the caravan site and actually went passed it and discovered we had found the wrong site, about two miles from the one we wanted. Eventually we arrived and I was able to take my bearings in the large static caravan. There was a bathroom and toilet at one end and a sitting room at the other with a passage connecting them. This passage doubled as a reasonably well appointed kitchen. Leading from this area were three bedrooms, one with a double bed and the other two with bunks. Some of the seats in the sitting room also converted to beds and I imagine that in a holiday brochure the caravan would be described as 'eight berth' but it was rather cramped with six of us.

As it was not the holiday season, the caravan had probably stood empty through the winter months and although all the heaters had been on at full blast since early afternoon, it wasn't very warm. I had a bath and put on some fresh clean clothes that Edna had brought for me before sitting down to what can only be described as a feast. There was not enough room on the table for all the food that Marjorie and Dorothy had prepared. Six healthy appetites made a significant inroad, but there was enough left to ensure that there would be no problems deciding what to have for lunch the next day. When the meal was over and the washing up done we sat talking and drinking coffee until someone noticed that there were people moving about outside. There seemed to be numbers of people all heading in the same direction and, being curious, we put our coats on and followed the flow. We soon realised that we were approaching a large clubroom from which we could hear music. Apparently there was a dance going on. People who belonged to Old Time and Sequence Dance Clubs were spending a week's holiday enjoying their pastime and they had brought with them their own band. In the foyer one could buy shoes, foot cream and other aids to their art. We were neither dressed for dancing nor in the mood to join them so we took a quiet stroll along the roads adjoining the site before returning to the caravan.

I needed to study my route for the next day and it was difficult to find anywhere to be alone in these conditions. I explained that it was necessary for me to find a little peace and quiet and why I needed it and I was left alone with my map. I felt that there were things that needed to be sorted out with the others, for example it was clear I could not return all this way for breakfast. Maurice and Douglas assured me that they would be with me tomorrow and would see to everything, all I had to think about was the walking. I was still dubious but I had to be satisfied at that.

My two helpers were not just brothers-in-law but also friends of many years standing. Maurice is the same age as me and as we had been childhood neighbours we had gone to school together and shared a desk, worked together and joined the Air Force at the same time. After Demob. we had worked together again for a while until circumstances sent us off in different directions but we always stayed in touch and had many friends and interests in common. Douglas is a few years younger and our acquaintance only goes back as far as 1947. He is unflappable and has a dry sense of humour and I find him very good company. I therefore knew I was in good hands.

Edna and I had been allocated the room with the double bed which was easily the biggest and most comfortable of any. We were all tired and in bed before eleven o'clock. Well, almost! Douglas moved in his bed and it collapsed tipping him onto the floor. The pandemonium that followed while we tried to sort things out as Douglas gave us his considered opinion about bunk beds ended with us all convulsed with laughter and as a result it seemed to take ages to get off to sleep.

Day Twenty seven

The little man in my clock told me rather formally that it was five fifty a.m. and I decided to get up quietly and make a cup of tea for the others in order to help them wake up. First of all I disturbed Edna when I got out of bed, then , on my way to the toilet, I kicked over the rubbish bin with a crash that was loud enough to wake half the people on the campsite. Then on the way back I managed to get the doors to the bedroom and bathroom jammed together so that I could neither open nor shut either of them and I was trapped in the bathroom. There was a crash for which I was not responsible and Dorothy put her head round their bedroom door to say, with tears of laughter running down her face, that Douglas' bed had collapsed again. Those who had been rudely awakened and come to try and rescue me from the bathroom deserted me and went to see what had happened. As far as I could make out the bed had folded trapping him in much the same way as a collapsed deck chair might, and his attempts to get free proved to be hilarious for the rest of them to watch. I remember thinking that it was a good thing we had no near neighbours with all this riotous behaviour before six o'clock in the morning. Eventually Douglas freed himself from the vicious bed and Maurice managed to untangle the door handles that were causing my imprisonment in the bathroom and some semblance of order returned.

It was cold and the three ladies returned to their warm beds while we turned up the heaters, put on warm clothes and made a hot drink. Everyone agreed that the mornings mayhem had all been my fault.

"When George wakes up, everyone wakes up!"

I have broad shoulders and accepted the blame.

After a hot drink and a light breakfast and with coffee and sandwiches packed, the three of us set off towards Appledore. The weather this morning was a great improvement on the previous one, dry, bright and cold. I did not mind the cold as I soon got warm when walking fast.

It was not yet half past seven as I set off along the road to Sampford Peverell and Tiverton. I could not help thinking about the chaos of the morning and wondering if I had been wise in my choice of helpers. I had been spoilt by the quiet consideration of my previous minders. I soon realised that I had nothing to worry about and that I was in Excellent hands. At a roundabout where the A373 crosses under the M5 on the way from Appledore to Sampford Peverell, I found Maurice waiting to ensure that I did not go astray. When I reached Tiverton, Douglas was standing by the roadside and led me to a nearby cafe where Maurice had already ordered tea and a plate of bacon sandwiches for each of us. This was a good and convenient solution to the problem of breakfast, there was no need to go off the route and there was no time lost.

Maurice walked, or rather hobbled because of his damaged ankle, through Tiverton with me, guiding me down a side road to cut a corner, the sort of thing I would not have risked on my own. Douglas drove through the town and picked up Maurice when I was safely on the A3072 to Crediton. The day was now warm and bright, a cuckoo constantly reminding us that it was spring. The need to concentrate and the threat from the proximity of the traffic were my constant companions but it was nevertheless a pleasure to walk through the Devon countryside.

After Tiverton the road crosses the River Exe then runs alongside it for two miles until at Bickleigh the river forks south towards Exeter while the road continues in a more westerly direction through Cadbury and Stockley Pomeroy to Crediton.

We had lunch at Crediton, stopping in a lay-by where there was a caravan from which a lady was serving drinks and snacks with which we could supplement our sandwiches. Maurice was completely taken aback when the lady refused to take any money and instead offered him a generous donation to put in the collecting tin. She said that she had suffered from cataracts which had been operated on and now she could see perfectly.

When I set off after lunch, Maurice came with me for a little way to make sure that I turned west on the A377 towards Copplestone. This was a straightforward piece of navigation and I could probably have managed it without help, but I have the principle that it is better to accept help when it may not be needed than to do without it when it is. As we walked I told him that the generosity of the lady at the catering caravan was typical of the kindness and support of the people I had met along the route.

My helpers were waiting for me at Copplestone to remind me to bear left on to the A3072 towards Bow and Okehampton. I told them that my target for that day was a place about seven miles from there near North Tawton where the B3215 forks left to Okehampton and suggested that they go on to there and I would see them at about four o'clock. They did not think it was a good idea to be that far away from me and I caught up with them twice more before the end of the day. As it turned out, they were right because the sky clouded and a steady drizzle meant that waterproofs were needed for the last three miles.

There was thirty miles to drive to the campsite at Westward Ho where we were to spend another night and along the winding roads the trip took an hour. The three ladies had thoroughly enjoyed their day. They had been to the beach and the harbour and of course the shops. They had ventured as far as Barnstaple where Edna had bought me a new pair of trainers as she had noticed that mine were completely worn out. I liked to wear them for the last few miles when the weather was fine. We had a cup of tea while we listened to the account of their day and then, while I got washed and changed, Maurice and Douglas attempted to repair Douglas' bed for despite many requests he refused to do a repeat performance of the show he had put on for us that morning.

After another enormous meal had been prepared and disposed of it was suggested that we pass the evening away by going for a walk round the harbour and then call at one of the local hostelries for a drink. It had been an easy day's walk and I wasn't at all tired but I made sure that before we went out I had time to myself to study the route for tomorrow. The ladies were eager to demonstrate their knowledge of the local geography and we went in two cars to a car park that they had discovered adjacent to the harbour. I was interested to see that there were quite large freighters docked there, one I think was Russian and the other Swedish.

It was cold and damp so we did not spend much time sightseeing and we soon put the second part of the plan into operation and found a quiet, warm and comfortable pub. We relaxed here until ten o'clock when we were all feeling tired. I am sure this was because we were in a warm atmosphere but everyone else seemed to think it was because I had woken them up so early that morning. We returned to the not so warm caravan and had a warm drink before going to bed. I was given the privilege of first use of the bathroom and on the way I moved the waste bin out of harms way so there would be no risk of my kicking it over again. We then witnessed the amazing sight of Douglas getting into bed. The sight of this large man folding himself gingerly into such a narrow and unstable bed was a feat worthy of the applause we gave him.

Day Twenty eight

I was up and dressed well before six and after successfully negotiating my way to the bathroom with a minimum of noise I had returned to the kitchen and filled the kettle and I was in the corridor when Maurice stepped out of his bedroom and I walked into him, tipping half the contents of the kettle over him and sending the lid clattering on to the floor. That plus Maurice's startled exclamation made sure that everyone else was awake to and I knew that I was in trouble again. The fact that it was not my fault made no difference and the general consensus was that I would make less noise and mess if they gave me a drum to beat at six o'clock in the morning to ensure that everyone was as awake as me!

At last the kettle was on and we set about trying to warm up the caravan. This time however, the gas heater defied all our efforts to get it going. For fifteen minutes or more each the men tried to persuade the clacking, clicking ignition system to work. Finally Dorothy, unable to stand the noise, came out of her bedroom, pushed us out of the way and with her very first effort got the fire going. Then without a word she returned to her bed.

It did not take long to have a quick bite to eat, make our preparations and set off. It was warmer in the car than in the caravan. Whether we took a shorter route back to my starting point or whether it just took less time I do not know but I was walking by five past seven. It was now Saturday 27th April and four weeks since I had left home to start this walk. I now had only one hundred and ten miles to go to complete it. This thought was in my mind as I set out on a cold, clear and bright morning along a quiet road through lovely countryside towards Okehampton which I reached in a little over an hour. Maurice was waiting their to escort me round Okehampton, past the castle and on to the A30, the road that would take me to Launceston, nineteen miles away. I had walked nine miles when Douglas met me and we went to a roadside cafe where once again Maurice had organised food and drinks. In this case the food consisted of hot dogs, not the sort of breakfast I had grown used to but it was food at the right time and I enjoyed it and the short break. As usual as soon as I had finished eating I was anxious to be on my way. I liked this system of stopping at roadside places to eat as there was no wasted time and we could eat when we were hungry. I don't think it would have been feasible however further north since there are not so many roadside catering places as there are on these holiday routes in the south.

We were to spend one more night at Westward Ho and Douglas said that they had asked the ladies to find somewhere to stay after that within reach of Land's End, perhaps near Newquay. He had asked Dorothy to look for somewhere saying that he didn't care what she found as long as it was warm and the beds did not collapse!

The walking was easy, the road was a dual carriageway with plenty of room for me to walk between the kerb and the solid white line that runs the length of the road and which served as some protection from the passing traffic as it was a demarcation point between their territory and mine. Through Bridestowe, Lewdown and Lifton before crossing the River Tamar a mile east of Launceston. Here we stopped for a drink and a sandwich. I had come twenty four miles and it wasn't quite one o'clock. I suggested that if I walked another six or seven miles and then finished for the day there may be time to do a couple of hours with collecting tins in the town. My conscience was telling me that I had not stopped to collect donations since leaving Shrewsbury. Maurice and Douglas agreed to go into Launceston and see what it was like. There was no risk of my getting lost on this part of the journey as it was just a matter of staying on the A30 as it skirted south of Launceston and continued towards Bodmin. However Bodmin was not on today's schedule and at half past two I met my faithful minders in a lay-by at Tregadillett. They called out to me as I was about to walk past and it was a while before I could make them out. They were sitting in deck chairs enjoying the sunshine besides a caravan Cafe and all they needed to complete the picture of the holidaymaker was to roll their trousers up to the knee and a knotted handkerchief on their heads. There was a chair and a cup of coffee ready for me and explained that although Launceston was a nice enough place, they thought it would be a waste of time trying to collect in the streets there as there were very few people about. The idea was that we should drive into the town in case they had missed a busier part of it and that I should make a decision about whether to spend time collecting or not. It was true that the place was almost deserted so we drove straight back to Westward Ho. arriving there at half past three.

The ladies were surprised to see us so early and even more surprised to learn that I had walked thirty miles that day. They had good news for us, they had been to the Tourist Information office and had been given the telephone number of someone who let out flats in Newquay. They had telephoned and made a provisional booking. As the flat was let on a weekly basis and we only needed it for four days they had left the decision for all of us to make. We agreed that it would be fine and hopefully more comfortable than the caravan.

I sat back and listened while everyone else sorted out the plans for the next day, happy to let them get on with it. They decided that Edna and Maurice would accompany me in the morning while Douglas, whose car was the larger of the two, would take Marjorie, Dorothy and the luggage to the flat. He would then see them settled in before coming to take over from Edna. I also heard the ladies had taken the washing to a laundrette during the day where the owner had asked them if they were on holiday. When he found out exactly why they were there, he had done the washing and ironing without charging them suggesting they could put the money it would have cost in the collecting tin, another £5.00 to boost the fund.

With the arrangements made it was time to eat. I had suggested eating out but no-one else was keen as there was plenty of food there and I think the women enjoyed the catering and they did a very good job of it. After we had eaten I did my route studying while the washing up was being done and then we sat for a while deciding what to do with the evening. Eventually we settled for a stroll down to the harbour, a quiet drink and a stroll back. I was not very enthusiastic as walking in the dark is no pleasure to me but the alternative was to stay in the caravan and it really was not warm enough to feel comfortable and relax. The weather this evening was much better than it had been the evening before and we were able to see more, or at least the others were. I can see very little in the dark and with the knowledge of what might happen if I strained my eyes by trying to hard to see, I let the others lead me around. We tried a different pub which was not so comfortable and we were soon on the way back. I was relieved to get to the caravan again. The walk back seemed to take ages and I was feeling tired. Distances walked in bad visibility always seem greater than they are. The only other noteworthy incident that night was the inevitable failure of the running repairs to Douglas' bed which once again collapsed.

Day Twenty nine

I was awake first the next morning and with the skill gained from two previous chaotic experiences managed to get washed and dressed, light the fire and make the tea without disturbing anyone. I checked the time by my clock and the little man's voice told me that it was five thirty two a.m. Still creeping about, I thought I would have some cereal and toast before waking the others with a cup of tea. I knew the cereals were kept in an overhead cupboard. I reached in and grasped the box with no problems but as I pulled it from the cupboard, two tins came with it and one, full of biscuits, hit the stainless steel sink with a noise like a bomb going off at that silent hour of the morning, and scattered biscuits and crumbs far and wide. The other tin hit me sharply on the ankle and I was hopping around oohing and aahing , holding my damaged ankle and grinding biscuits underfoot when everyone emerged from their various doorways chorusing uncomplimentary remarks. Someone, I don't remember who, took my arm and with a remarkable lack of gentleness marched me into the sitting area and sat me down out of the way until the chaos was sorted out. I was not allowed to move until my breakfast was ready. While I was eating I was treated to Douglas doing a parody of what he had seen when he got out of bed that morning...me hopping about, holding one foot in both hands and stating in no uncertain terms what I though of people who jam things into cupboards. This episode was funnier because Douglas was having trouble straightening his back after a night creased up in his broken bed. The laughter simmered down and Edna was treated to a great deal of sympathy from the other family members for putting up with me all the time!

We started to prepare for the day. We were able to pack most of our luggage into our car and this did not take long. Edna and Maurice were then told not to wait to tidy up but to get me out of the way as soon as possible. Its a good job I've got a thick skin!

It was 28th April, a lovely, calm sunny Sunday when, at half past seven, I started walking. I reckoned that there were seventy four more miles to go until I reached Land's End and if I was to get there by the end of the month, I had two and a half days to cover the distance. The tin that had hit my ankle that morning had knocked off a bit of skin but had done no lasting damage and caused me no inconvenience at all. The A30 was easy going for me, dual carriageway for the most part, undulating through pleasant scenery. There was not a lot of traffic although what there was seemed to be going fast. When I next met up with Edna and Maurice they were parked in a lay-by near Altarnum. Edna looked pale and upset. She had been watching me approaching with the traffic racing past and had convinced herself that I was in mortal danger from each and every one of the vehicles, especially the larger ones which made the car shake as they passed it. From then on she refused to look back along the road for me. I was thankful that she had not been with us on some of the narrower and much busier roads.

Edna was surprised when after a few seconds break I set off again, she had expected me to have a ten minute break at each stopping point. I did have a rest at the next stop, which was at a roadside cafe two miles further on where I enjoyed an enormous bacon sandwich that Maurice had bought for me. The respite was nevertheless brief because I wanted to take full advantage of this perfect weather for walking. I had been told that the forecast was for rain by late afternoon and that it would continue for several days.

An hour later as I pressed on, being all too aware that this weather was too good to last I was listening to what I think must have been the bubbling call of a female cuckoo. For the last two hundred miles the cuckoo call had been my almost constant companion but earlier in the year among bird songs played on a tape from the Shropshire Talking Newspaper had been one of the female cuckoo and now I thought that that was what I could hear. I was wishing that I could ask someone to confirm it when my reverie was disturbed by the hooting of a car horn and shouting from a window as a car went past. I did not have long to wait to find out what all the noise had been about. When I reached the next lay-by my daughter, son-in-law, their two children and a young French woman who was staying with them at the time all greeted me enthusiastically. They had driven that morning from their home in Ringwood, Hampshire to cheer me in this last stage of my endeavour. Their young French visitor had been keen to come and see this grandfather who she probably thought of as quite mad!

The children had apparently told anyone who would listen about what their Granddad was doing and the eldest, a lad of twelve wanted to walk some of the way with me. I was not keen as I thought it was too dangerous and also that it might slow me down. In the event I need not have worried, he very sensibly kept as near to the kerb as possible and during the three miles that he walked in front of me he kept up as fast a speed as I wanted.

Those three miles brought us to Bodmin where Edna and Maurice were waiting in a lay-by. Our daughter, Marilyn and her husband Peter were with them, amused by the fact that Edna refused to look along the road to see if we were coming. After a noisy and chaotic ten minutes I set off again, this time alone. Alexis, my grandson had decided that he had done his stint and anyway they had left their home in a hurry and had not had much to eat so they were going off to get a meal and said they would catch up with us again later.

It was a little early for me to stop for lunch and I wanted to get on. The interruptions were wasting this precious walking weather. Everyone was in Carnival mood and I did not want to spoil the party atmosphere so I began to walk on. They were all so busy laughing and chatting that I don't think they noticed.

After a while first the car with my daughter and her family passed me, then Edna and Maurice, both of them tooting the horn so that I knew they were in front of me. It was near Lanival that I met up with Edna and Maurice again and this time it was for a lunch break. I made this as brief as I decently could and I was soon on my way again leaving Edna and Maurice to wait for the others to catch up with them. I had not gone far before what seemed like a whole convoy of cars tooted their way past me and when I reached the next lay-by there were three cars in it. Douglas had joined the others and he was explaining where the flat was. When he was asked what the flat was like, he grimaced, shrugged and said that it was bigger and warmer than the caravan and left it at that. I ascertained that Douglas was taking over from Edna and I set off again. I had walked over twenty miles so far that day which was good but I felt flustered and a little irritated by the frequent interruptions to my walking rhythm. I soon got into my stride again and I heard the toots as the three cars went passed, two of them heading for Newquay and the other, with Douglas in I knew would be waiting for me two or three miles along the road.

This section of the road was being straightened or made into a dual carriageway and consequently was plagued with road works of the worst kind for me. Three times that day I lost the road when the edge that I was following ended in a bank of earth. On the first occasion after clambering over a mound of earth I stepped into a trench about three feet deep landing heavily and awkwardly on my right leg sending a spasm of pain through my knee. Climbing out I found myself in a kind of no mans land. The scarred landscape, the trenches and the great, silent earth moving machines feeding my imagination. From a high point I could see traffic on the road a hundred yards away and painfully and carefully made my way towards it wondering how I could have gone so far astray.

Once again I had a problem with my knee. Surely I wasn't going to be stopped so near to my objective? I tried to put any negative thoughts out of my mind and gradually the pain eased and my spirits rose. The sun had disappeared behind some threatening clouds but it was still quite warm and pleasant. I had learned my lesson and on the next to occasions when I ran out of road, I retraced my steps and wove my way around the red and white witches' hats. At least as it was Sunday there were no working men and machines to dodge.

At the end of the section of road works, Douglas was waiting for me and apologised for not coming to my aid sooner. The roadworks and 'no parking' signs had made it impossible for him to stop before this. I was pleased that he had not noticed that I was walking a little stiffly as I'm sure he would have felt guilty though it was not his fault. I had begun to realise how very responsible my minders felt towards me.

We were near to Indian Queens and my target for the day was four miles on at Carland Cross. However with my concern for my knee uppermost in my mind I suggested that it might be better to stop at Summercourt as there was a road from there direct to Newquay. This would be two miles short of my objective but I had still walked over thirty miles that day, and with only forty four left to do I thought I had earned an early finish.

It was four o'clock when I reached Summercourt and fifteen minutes later we arrived at Fistral Bay, Newquay. Douglas drove into an attractive courtyard where we were greeted by Maurice and Peter and escorted to a large, warm and welcoming ground floor flat. The flat had three bedrooms one of which had en-suite facilities. This was allocated to Edna and me, not, it was made clear out of philanthropic motives, but in an attempt to keep me out of the way for a bit longer in the morning. There was a separate bathroom, a kitchen and a large sitting room with patio doors leading to a paved area and garden. There were tables and chairs outside and if it had been warm enough I would have liked to sit there and look at the view which was breathtaking. We overlooked Fistral Bay with Newquay and the promontory of Towan Head on the right and the ruggedly beautiful Cornish coastline on the left leading to Kelsey Head and Holywell Bay. I remembered camping holidays at Holywell when the children were young, especially the one when every tent on the site was blown down in a gale. Ours had been torn in the process and we had taken it to a sail maker in Perranporth to be repaired so that we could continue with our holiday.

The rain that had been threatening for the last hour or two was now falling as steady drizzle but that did not bother us in that comfortable place where, even with eleven of us, it did not seem overcrowded. I took a bath and then spent a while studying what I hoped would be my last full day of walking, working out where I wanted to finish in order to leave me with just the right distance to walk on the last day. I had decided to try to reach Land's End by two o'clock, as that meant that I would have completed the walk within thirty days. This made it neat and tidy in my mind. To do this I decided that, ideally, I would like to get west of St. Ives and within twelve miles of my goal when I finished walking on the following day. There was one thing bothering me however, my right knee that I had hurt when falling into the trench. I had landed foot first but heavily and awkwardly twisting the knee. It was the same knee that I had damaged earlier in the walk but it was not the same type of injury. There was no swelling or bruising just an ache and a feeling of lack of stability.

The studying took quite a while and I did not hurry, enjoying the peace of my bedroom compared with the noise and hilarity that was going on in the sitting room. Shortly after I emerged Marilyn and her family and friend set off on their long drive back to Hampshire. I had been pleased to see them, but I was not in the most sociable frame of mind and it was good to enjoy the comparative tranquillity of the company of the six adults. There was no temptation to go out that evening. We ate a meal cooked by the ladies and the men did the washing up. For the next three hours or so we relaxed discussing our plans and generally putting the world right. Unusually for me I told them my thoughts about how and when I would complete the walk. I did not mention my knee.

Since joining me, Edna had taken over the task of making any necessary telephone calls, keeping the Charity and other members of the family informed of my progress. Among the people she called was Harry Field who expressed a wish to join me in walking the last few miles. I was happy to agree, suggesting that he could stay at the flat for a night if he wanted to, there was a bed-settee in the sitting room and it would not be a problem. Harry, therefore, was going to drive down and join us tomorrow. As it was Sunday there was no point in trying to contact anyone at the Charity Headquarters that day so Edna said she would telephone in the morning in case they wanted to arrange for anyone to be a t Land's End to meet us.

I would rather have liked to keep quiet about the finish especially as I was aware that forty four miles could be a long way with a game knee but since no-one knew of my niggling worry and I did not intend to say anything about it, I had to let the organisation go on. At half past ten I decided that it was my bedtime. There was some talk of a concerted attempt to keep me awake in the hope that I might oversleep, but Edna scotched this plan by telling them that I would still wake up early and probably be twice as clumsy and noisy if I had not had enough sleep. Anyway, it had been a long day for all of us and they were tired too.

Day Thirty

I opened my eyes in the morning and listened to the sound of the rain on the window. I pressed the clock button to be told that it was five thirty five a.m. For a fleeting minute I was tempted to have another half hour in bed but the thought that this was the last full day of the walk overcame this and a cold wash soon had me wide awake. I put the light on in the kitchen, filled the kettle and set it to boil and returned to the bedroom to get dressed. Edna was awake but keeping her eyes closed hoping to have a cup of tea to help her wake up. The kettle boiled but I couldn't find any tea. After a vain search I asked Edna where it was in a stage whisper. She poked her head into the kitchen and said

"It's over there" my reply was an irritated

"Where is 'there'?" Up, down, left or right mean something to me but 'there' is no help at all. Edna, who is not a t her best before six in the morning, stormed into the kitchen, pulled out a tin clearly marked 'Tea' and then began to laugh as she opened it to find that it was full of sugar. Eventually we found the right one, but of course by this time we had disturbed the others. Maurice was the first to appear, grumbling that this was what happened when the Jones's were given the bridal suite. Douglas soon followed and it was not long before we had had drinks and cereals, stocked up with flasks of coffee and were on our way. We were not bothering to prepare sandwiches since there were plenty of eating places on the route. We left the flat at seven o'clock and a quarter of an hour later I was walking, head down into a strong wind, waterproofs zipped right up against the driving rain. The road was wet and muddy, a result of the still frequent road works. I was finding even the slightest uphill gradient difficult and a sore test of my damaged knee. Thirty two miles was going to seem a long way today. From Summercourt through Carland Cross and Zelah I struggled. Twice I was helped by road builders who were dressed in luminous waterproofs like me and were probably just as uncomfortable. At the sight of my white stick they came and guided me through the forest of equipment and cones and one of them even gave me £1.00 to put in my tin.

Between Blackwater and Redruth Douglas was waiting to guide me into a roadside cafe. It was half past ten and we were all hungry. They had been looking for somewhere suitable to stop since nine o'clock but as everyone knows when you do not want to stop and eat there is a cafe to mark every mile, and when you do, they magically disappear. Douglas and Maurice confirmed that in spite of the bad weather and adverse conditions, I had come twelve miles in three and a quarter hours. I took off my mud-spattered waterproofs, dried my feet, put on fresh socks and boots and settled down to enjoy the large well-cooked breakfast that had been organised for me. The extra effort I had put in had given me an appetite. An intake of food and the knowledge that I was making good time put new heart into me. The rain had relented by the time I set off again at eleven and there was now a light drizzle. In my zipped up waterproofs I was uncomfortably warm but if I unzipped them the strong headwind blew the dampness at me. My knee was fine on the level or downhill but was painful on the uphill stretches and the steeper the hill the more it hurt.

I continued along the A30 bypassing Redruth and Camborne. The road is fairly straight and well surfaced and another time I might have enjoyed it but on this day with the wind blowing the drizzle in my face and my leg troubling me, I was not s happy man. My knee seemed to be getting worse and the dreadful thought occurred to me that if it swelled up badly I would probably not be able to finish. No-one else knew that I had a problem and I wanted it to stay my secret. I did not want Edna worrying or any advice no matter how well meant. I was sure that I would have been told to see a doctor or rest my knee for a day or two and I intended to complete the walk the next day even if I had to hop the last few miles and nothing was going to stop me now I had got this far.

After Camborne the road reverted to single carriageway which held the water better, or so I thought, the quality of spray from passing vehicles had definitely improved and once or twice it had almost a solid feel to it. Maurice and Douglas were very concerned, hardly letting me out of their sight. Perhaps they suspected that something was wrong though nothing was said directly. It was suggested that at one o'clock when we stopped for a break and a coffee that we call it a day and hope for better weather tomorrow. We were then at Connor Downs which is about twenty miles from Land's End and seven or eight miles short of my target for that day. For a moment I was tempted to agree to the proposition but the thought that my leg might get worse over night helped me to decide to go on and think again in about an hour's time.

I set off again and in about a mile I found them waiting for me at Phillack on the eastern side of Hayle. Douglas had on his waterproofs and walked with me through Hayle and as far as Canonstown, leaving me only when he was sure I was on the right road. If the car had been with us then I think I would have stopped but Douglas was intending to walk back over a mile to where it was parked so I carried on. The rain had almost stopped but waterproofs were still needed because of the spray and anyway it was too late to stop and take them off for it would make no difference to my progress now. I reached a lay-by where my road turned west along the coast towards Penzance and another went east to nearby Marazion. I could just about make out St. Michael's Mount through the cloud and mist.

This was one of the few occasions on the whole walk when I was really tired but nevertheless I was within thirteen miles of Land's End and very pleased to have reached this point. A few minutes later the car pulled up and I wearily pulled off my leggings and jacket. I was soaked in sweat and thought longingly of climbing into and soaking in a hot bath when we got back to the flat. The half hour it took to drive back seemed endless.

Harry Field had arrived and was waiting with the ladies to greet us. They were surprised at how far I had travelled that day in such difficult conditions, and I was glad they did not know the full story. I had covered thirty one miles, and everyone cheered when I said that there was only another twelve or thirteen miles to go. I planned to have a real rest and start walking at about ten o'clock which would leave me with an easy four hours of walking. I wanted to arrive at Land's End at two o'clock as that would correspond to the time when I had started off, thirty days before.

A quick cup of tea and then into the bath. The water was hot when I got in but I soaked for so long that it had gone quite cool by the time I got out. As I lay in the bath, more tired physically than at any other time on the walk, my thoughts wandered back to the start, to the breakdown of the caravanette, the snowstorm on Drumochter, the day I left Monmouth with an aching head and eyes and a score of other incidents along the way. Despite the tiredness I felt good, there was no pain from my knee, no cuts or blisters on my feet and I was convinced that nothing could now prevent me from reaching my goal. I now noticed that five of my toenails had gone black. Three on one foot and two on the other. These later came off but caused no discomfort.

When I rejoined the others I felt much better with fresh dry clothes and a delicious smell from the kitchen encouraging my appetite. Edna had telephoned the Fight For Sight people and told them of my expected time of arrival at Land's End. They said that they had organised a reception and arranged for Edna and I to stay overnight at the Hotel there. The evening meal was a cheerful one. Good food and good company in warm comfortable surroundings. Harry in particular was pleased and excited at the prospect of walking with me to the finish of a journey that he had helped to start. After the meal and while the washing up was being done I went off to study my route for the last time. This time there was no danger of my getting lost but I wanted to know where I was as I went along so that I could time my arrival correctly.

I returned to the sitting room with impeccable timing just as all the tidying up was finished and coffee was being served. This was the prelude to a very enjoyable evening. The persistent rain discouraged any thoughts of going out and indeed made the flat seem even more cosy by contrast. As the evening wore on my attempts at conversation grew less and the effort of keeping my eyes open grew greater. I decided it was time for me to go to bed and accompanied by dire threats of what might happen to me if I woke anyone up before half past seven the next morning.

The Final day

The first time I pressed the button on my clock it was six a.m. The second time it was a quarter past and the third time it was half past. Then, threats or no threats, I could lie in bed no longer. I got up, washed and dressed and made a pot of tea. I poured myself a cup and sat down on the settee to drink it, forgetting that Harry was using it as a bed, and sat on him! Instantly awake he sat up sending me and my tea flying. I did a juggling act and managed to save about half the contents of my cup. The other half going over either him or me and being hot enough to cause a noisy reaction. People appeared, it seemed from everywhere, concerned at first and then when they realised that there was no real harm done they disappeared as quickly as they had come only pausing to say something uncomplimentary about my early morning performances. Even taking them a cup of tea did little to change their pre-seven o'clock opinion of me.

By the time Harry had drunk our tea and had some cereal the place was alive and a cooked breakfast was being prepared and the table laid. A whole chorus of voices refused my offer to help and I was ordered to stay where I was and my food would be brought to me. Breakfast over, preparations were made for the day. Flasks of coffee were made and Edna packed an overnight bag for the two of us. It had been decided that we would all set off at the same time and meet at the point near Marazion where the walking would begin. After photographs had been taken and Harry and I were on our way the ladies would go into Penzance to do some shopping and rejoin us again on the road somewhere near Sennen at about one o'clock prior to the very last few miles.

We left the flat at half past nine and reached the starting point shortly before ten. The weather was showing a considerable improvement on the previous day, the wind had dropped and though it was dark and overcast, it was not raining. After an extended photograph session Harry and I set off. First Edna tooted as she drove off with the ladies into Penzance and then I heard Maurice and Douglas pass. I felt good as there was no discomfort at all from my knee. Harry chatted as we strode along the A30 in high spirits. Through Penzance ,I knew that we were now exactly ten miles from Land's End. One more mile and I would be on the last one percent of the journey. I mentioned this and Harry reminded me of the time what seemed like ages before when we had reached Wick on the first day and I said proudly that I had done two percent of the journey already.

This part of the road was surprisingly busy although at Drift the road

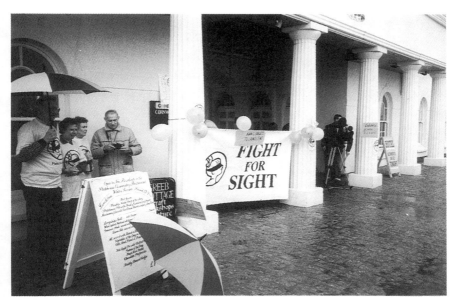

The Reception Commitee

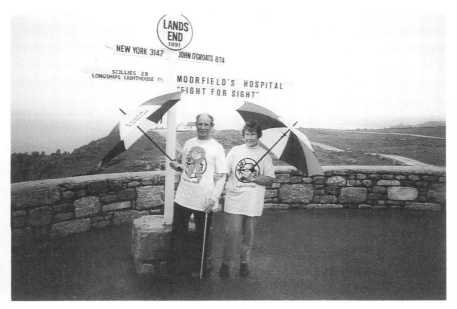

Home and Dry

149

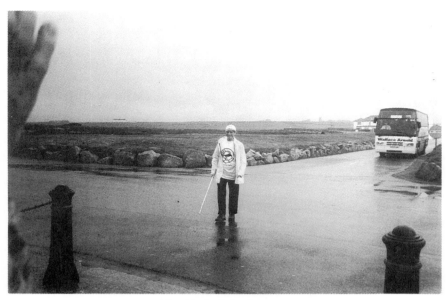

The End of the Journey

forked and much of the traffic turned south on the B3283 while we continued towards Sennen on the A30. We were travelling at a good speed and I reckoned that we would have an hour to spare so when we next caught up with Maurice and Douglas I suggested that they find a place to stop near where the B3306 forks right towards St. Just. I expected to reach there at about half past twelve.

We were passing fields with cauliflower growing and we noticed also large wire mesh bins at the roadside with cauliflower in. We noticed that they were unusually big, much larger than any I had grown. Harry pointed out a particularly handsome specimen and I turned in order to try to see it. The next second I was in a heap on the floor. A momentary lapse of concentration and I had stepped off the road into a depression and the result of my fall was a strain of something in my thigh. Harry was very contrite, blaming himself for distracting my attention but of course it was not his fault. I had spent a lot of time training myself to avoid being distracted and anyway there was no serious damage even though it did cause me to limp for a while. It merely served to emphasise how much safer it was for me in general to walk alone.

We arrived at the junction as I had said, at half past twelve. There we met with the others, as by this time the ladies had also arrived. It had started to drizzle and we were content to sit in the car and let the time pass. I was able to clean my muddy hands and brush my clothes with a little help from my friends. After about five minutes, Maurice and the ladies went off for some pre-conceived purpose that I had not been informed about. At quarter past one we started on the final two miles. Douglas drove past to join the others and await our arrival. The drizzle was a nuisance, too wet to ignore but not bad enough to warrant putting all my waterproof gear on. I compromised by wearing just my coat. After passing through Sennen we turned right on the approach to Land's End and I was met by a man who said he was from Southwest Television and that he wanted to film my arrival and would I wait a minute or two while he got back to his cameras. Harry went on and after a short while I followed to walk the last two hundred yards towards the cameras and the six members of my fan club who had put up a large banner declaring 'The Fight For Sight' decorated with many balloons. There were two coach loads of tourists standing nearby looking bemused and no doubt wondering what all the fuss was about. My party started to cheer as I walked towards them then I heard a shout of alarm from Douglas who ran towards me but he was too late to prevent me sprawling over a chain fence across the entrance to the area. So, in this undignified manner, the walk was completed.

The camera man asked me to walk the last bit again without the trip over and I obliged. We then followed a young woman who had introduced herself as the Public Relations Manager for the Land's End complex to the famous signpost for the obligatory photographs. This had been arranged and paid for by the Charity, but it was all that had been arranged by them. No-one knew anything about the promised overnight stop at the hotel and I later discovered that the television people had arrived because my son-in-law had telephoned them with the story and not through any efforts by the Charity on my behalf.

Edna wanted to send about fifty postcards to people bearing the Land's End postmark. We were told that this was not possible since cards sent from there would have a Sennen postmark. The young woman offered to stamp each of the cards with a rubber stamp having a picture of the lighthouse and the name Land's End. This was easier said than done, the offices were a shambles as they were being re-organised and redecorated and everything was in boxes under dust sheets. There were no other staff there, and our helper had only been employed there for a week. It took her a while to unearth the stamp but she found it eventually and duly stamped the cards and our log. We then joined the others and found a restaurant for a light snack before we set off back to the flat in Newquay.

Harry was by far the most thrilled, he thought that I had achieved something great and could not understand why I was not turning cartwheels in my delight. To tell the truth there was a sense of anti-climax. It had not been as difficult or as arduous as I had expected. I was not tired or exhausted and did not feel that I had done anything exceptional enough to warrant a lot of fuss. The people who had really worked hard and deserved much of the credit were my minders. They had had the constant worry and trouble of looking after me, had put up with my whims and wishes and made the whole thing easy for me.

It was decided that we should go out for a celebration dinner. It was to be my treat so that I could in some small way thank these good friends for all they had done for me. When Maurice and Douglas had said to me that all I had to do was the walking and that they would see to everything else, they had spoken the truth and were as good as their word, organising transport, food lodgings and all incidentals. Before we went out someone put on the television and we waited to see if the film of my arrival was shown. There it was, right at the end of the local news, a few words, a brief flash of colour and it was over, far too quickly for me to adjust my eyes to see it properly. This brief moment of fame however added to our high spirits as we prepared for our evening out.

The party mood continued all evening. The restaurant was excellent and supplied us with good food and wine. It was a happy, noisy group which returned to the flat at the end of that memorable day.

The Aftermath

We had had an offer of help from a lady in Exeter if we wanted to do some collecting there and we decided to do this on our way home. I got up at half past six, made some tea and had breakfast, this time without disturbing anyone else. I then took everyone else a cup of tea again without breaking or spilling anything. Edna and I left for Exeter at quarter to nine. Harry left for home at the same time but the others were staying for another day or two. Edna had arranged to meet our volunteer helper in Exeter town centre at two o'clock.

It was a damp and miserable day, not good conditions for fund raising. Nevertheless we did well, collecting over £100 .00 in an hour and a half. One young man asked about the walk and how long it had taken me. He said that he had done the route by bicycle and it had taken him a week. He gave generously and then returned a little while later to donate even more. At this point Mary, the lady who had so kindly helped us this afternoon went to collect her children from school and after a reviving hot drink we set off for Bristol where we were to stay overnight.

I thought Edna would enjoy a night with Mrs. Truscott at Pilning and I had telephoned to book a room. Edna was as impressed as Eric and I had been and I learned that Eric had also stayed there on his way home. The evening was dry and clear and Edna and I walked the short distance along the lane to the local inn where we had a meal and spent a pleasant evening. On the way back Edna picked up a screwed up piece of paper. I asked her what it was and she said she thought it was money. Sure enough it was a £20.00 note. I was amazed. At night everything is so black to me that I can't imagine anyone being able to see anything, let alone recognise a piece of paper on the ground. Another contribution to the fund.

The following morning, after breakfast, we said good-bye to Mrs. Truscott and set off for home, over the Severn Bridge and along that lovely Wye Valley road, through Monmouth, Hereford and Ludlow. The sun was shining and it was a glorious spring day to welcome me home.

There was still much to be done, money collected and letters answered. The walk was complete and although the light at the end of my tunnel will never get any nearer, I hope the money raised will go some way to helping others to Fight for Sight. The walk, approximately nine hundred miles, had taken thirty days. That time included one day without walking and three when I only walked for half a day. The amount raised when everything was eventually collected was over £7,500.

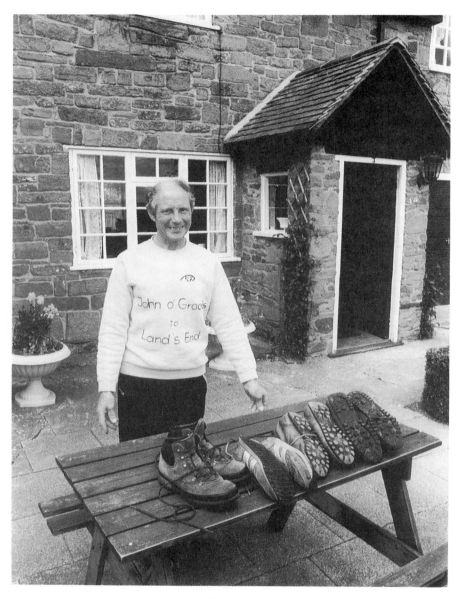

Worn out

I had met many friendly, helpful, generous people along the way. I knew that I had been fortunate in being able to count on Edna's organising ability, my dedicated group of minders for whom no amount of thanks and praise would be adequate, a supportive family and friends and good health.

My black toenails came off and my knee gave out on me while doing a strenuous hill walk later in the year, but since then I have walked in the Austrian Alps and backpacked from Mallaig to Montrose on the Route of the Ultimate Challenge without any ill-effects from it.

Many of the details of the walk were recorded en route on my Philip's pocket memo, others were laboriously written in my own form of shorthand but most of it came back to me as I mentally retraced my steps. I feel sure that some of the places and events I have described may seem entirely different to another clear-sighted observer but I have tried to describe as truthfully as possible the journey and happenings as they appeared to me.